The White Paper and Beyond

Proceedings of a National Conference on the White Paper *Working for Patients*, held 31 January 1990 at the Royal College of Physicians, London, and organized by the North West Thames Regional Health Authority in conjunction with the Faculty of Public Health Medicine, the Institute of Health Service Management and by courtesy of the Royal College of Physicians, London.

The White Paper and Beyond

One Year On

Edited by

E.J. Beck

Lecturer and Senior Registrar

St Mary's Hospital Medical School

and

S.A. Adam

Public Health Director

North West Thames Regional Health Authority

Oxford • New York • Tokyo

OXFORD UNIVERSITY PRESS

1990

Oxford University Press, Walton Street, Oxford OX2 6DP

Oxford New York Toronto
Delhi Bombay Calcutta Madras Karachi
Petaling Jaya Singapore Hong Kong Tokyo
Nairobi Dar es Salaam Cape Town
Melbourne Auckland

and associated companies in
Berlin Ibadan

Oxford is a trade mark of Oxford University Press

Published in the United States
by Oxford University Press, New York

British Library Cataloguing in Publication Data
The White Paper and beyond.
1. Great Britain Health Services
I. Beck, E.J. II, Adam, S.A.
362.10941
ISBN 0-19-262048-7
ISBN 0-19-261978-0

Library of Congress Cataloging in Publication Data
The White Paper and beyond : one year on / edited by E.J. Beck and S.A. Adam
Includes index.
1. National Health Service (Great Britain)–Congresses.
2. Medical policy–Great Britain–Congresses. 3. Public health–Great Britain–Congresses. I. Beck, Eduard J., 1955-
II. Adam, S . A . (Sheila A.)
RA412.5.G7W45 1990 362.1'0941–dc20 90-14239
ISBN 0-19-262048-7

Typeset by Cotswold Press Ltd
Printed in Great Britain by
Biddles Ltd, Guildford and King's Lynn

'I really like the hospital in the evening' Tahara had told him once. 'In the evening there's a light burning in every one of the hospital windows. It makes it look like a gigantic boat floating on the sea at night. And behind each of those windows, children are being born, and people are dying. They're all waging a battle against disease, the enemy of mankind. At times like that I always think that a doctor is someone who helps these people.'

Shusaku Endo
When I whistle

Acknowledgement

The Conference was only made possible through the combined efforts of numerous individuals from all organizations involved. From within North West Thames RHA we are grateful to all those individuals who provided their support, especially Jonathan Street, Annabel Brown, and the Registrars and Senior Registrars from the Department of Public Health. We are, however, particularly indebted to Jill Musgrove and Jane Savory for their invaluable assistance.

London E.J.B
March 1990 S.A.A

Contents

1

Welcome

DR SHEILA ADAM

We are here celebrating a first birthday and in many ways it has been a fairly typical first year. The White Paper has certainly made a lot of noise, it has been very demanding of people's time, and very disruptive to normal life. People have lost a lot of sleep over it, and I think, perhaps most interestingly, it has challenged a lot of our accepted wisdom, or certainly our accepted ways of doing things.

A lot of the discussion about the White Paper, because of pressures of time and pressures of other work, has tended to focus on some of the more mechanistic issues: organizational change, the purchaser/provider split, new funding arrangements including capitation funding, and different working relationships encompassed within the issue of contracts. We will certainly be touching on all of those issues here, but we also hope to look at some of the areas which we believe the White Paper could ensure. First, improved health status through health needs assessment, service option appraisal, and monitoring outcomes for both individuals and populations. Second, the opportunity to improve the quality of services with explicit quality standards and a shared professional and management commitment to quality. And third, new ways of working which value staff and which will include a shared sense of purpose not only within the Health Service but also with the other agencies on which we depend and with the communities for which we provide health care.

2

The White Paper: an overview
(Or: Fear and flattery on the campaign trail)

DR GREG PARSTON

I am both flattered and frightened to be here this morning: flattered because as someone who is not particularly known to be a friend of the White Paper, I am being asked to help celebrate the first year of its progress. It is quite an honour and I am happy with that, but it brings with it quite a responsibility.

I am also fearful because I know that someone who is invited to open an event such as this is really meant to soften things up. I do not really know that I have the ideas of the Kleins, the Kennys, the Culyers, or the Cunninghams to share with you—and so I am a bit frightened.

Fright brings with it another responsibility and that is that you do not tell people what they do not want to hear. So, I have decided that I should try to combine my fear and my flattery to try and steer a middle course. I do not know whether that means I am not going to tell you what you want to hear, or whether I am going to tell you what you do not want to hear. Indeed, I would like—with apologies to Hunter Thompson—to sub-title my talk 'Fear and Flattery on the Campaign Trail'.

An overview of the White Paper is quite difficult to provide. It is not like flying over the Eiffel Tower on its 101st birthday and taking an overview of that construction. It is much more dynamic; things are in flux. Dick Beckhard, an organization consultant, taught me a few years ago a method of organizational change called the 'helicopter ride' in which you try to position yourself above the changes that are being made. You pull yourself up further and further away and look down on the many forces that are taking place. It seems unclear to me that we can pull ourselves high enough above the White Paper to really get a good understanding of what all the forces are. As I tried to think about what the overview could be, I thought that getting an overview of the White Paper is like getting an overview of the recent South African cricket tour. What were we looking at? The game? The fact that there was not a very big audience there or that there were more police than audience or that there were more demonstrators than police? Or the system of apartheid around which this whole thing was being played? The White Paper poses the same sorts of problems for the helicopter pilot. What are we looking at? The purchaser/provider split? The doctors and clinical professionals who are part of the game? The Department of Health which is either guiding or policing events? The political debate in Parliament and outside? Or the market ideology which is really driving it? Any one of these elements could take 20 minutes or the whole day. Rather than trying to take a look at the overview of all events, what I have decided to do is to take a look at how the whole thing feels one year on. What does it feel like to be in the middle of the White Paper work? What does it feel like to have the policing, guiding, or debate going on?

A year ago, or a little less than a year ago, it felt panicky and confusing. Yet, at the same time, there was a spirit of initiative. Now there have been dozens of working papers and re-working papers. There have been literally hundreds of visits to market health services. I have friends at the Harvard Community Health Plan who told me that if I arranged one more visit there, I would be socially ostracized for ever! There were thousands of preparatory meetings, which none of us later can admit have happened. What does it feel like? It feels like panic, confusion, and initiative. It feels like the same thing. It feels like people are still racing to get ahead of a game they do not know. It feels like people are still very confused and it feels like there are still some people who are trying to exercise a spirit of initiative and maybe a little bit of leadership in this whole thing.

I do not think that I can do a lot about the panic. If you are a unit general manager who has seven weeks in front of you before you have to put your business plan together, there is nothing I am going to say which is going to allay the feeling of panic. Good luck!

Maybe though, through the course of the day, with the Kleins, the Kennys, the Culyers, and the Cunninghams, we will be able to enthuse a bit more of the spirit of initiative. A bit more of taking the lead, a bit more of putting on the agenda the new issues that Sheila Adam mentioned. In order to help do that, I thought that what I would try to focus on is the confusion and the lack of clarity that I see surrounding the changes that have been occurring over the last year.

One year ago, there was a great debate amongst people who were observing the changes about whether the White Paper was about *what* is to be done or *how* it is to be done. That debate still rages. Is the Department of Health telling us what to do and letting us get on with how to do it or is it in fact telling us how to do things and being as prescriptive as usual?

The debate around what and how over the year, to give the debate its due, has itself given form to new substantive confusions. That is, we are more confused now about certain substantive issues than about the what and the how. We are confused about what appears to be the re-emergence of hospitals. Friends, who I thought valued the comprehensiveness and continuity of care in the NHS as its most important features, are now talking about those days being over: 'The hospitals are back; let's start focusing on the hospitals.'

Others are much more confused and are saying, 'Wait a minute! What about community care? What about the fact that there is not just one White Paper but three? What about the fact that the incentives on local authorities and on health authorities are perverse and are leaving a big gap? What are we going to do about that confusion? What are we going to do about that big hole?'

A third confusion surrounds what is happening in primary care. What is happening with GP budgets? Are we being told what to do or are we being told how to do it? Can we really, honestly believe that GPs can be given budgetary responsibilities for providing care when they do not have statutory responsibilities for the health of the people to whom they are providing that care? Do we really believe that District Health

Authorities are going to let GPs buy services from hospitals with whom they do not contract? The district health authorities, in fact, have the statutory responsibility for the health of the population. Are we really talking about restricting GP referrals? I do not think anybody is willing to bite that bullet before the election and so we are lost in the confusion of what is happening in primary care as much as we are lost in the confusion of what is happening in community care, and what is happening in hospital care.

But all of this confusion continues to surround the questions: 'What are we doing?' and 'How are we doing it?'. I have argued for a year now that the bigger question is: 'Why is all this happening? Why are we doing this?' I do not have an answer to that but I think we need an answer. I would like to examine two possibilities, not from our point of view but from the point of view of the people who are either guiding or policing this.

The two people who I would like to take a look at are The Secretary of State for Health, Kenneth Clarke, and an imaginary Chancellor called Major Lawson. Mr Clarke might say that this whole thing is about the purchaser/provider split, building in market incentives, trying to get people to understand better how they can more effectively and efficiently purchase resources, services, and health if they are left to do so in a marketplace. How are we going to do that? That is up to you. If we give Mr Clarke the benefit of the doubt, his 'why?' is better health. I would have said some time ago that his 'why?' was his own political career but we have read in the newspapers recently that Conservative back-benchers are saying that what is left of Mr Clarke's political career is his memoirs, so I think we have to change our perspective on that. Let us give Mr Clarke the benefit of the doubt and say that why these changes are happening for him is to try to secure better health. The 'What?' is about the purchaser/provider split or the introduction of market economy and health care and 'How?' should be determined by people at the local level. That is one point of view.

Another point of view might be the Major Lawson point of view. Major Lawson is also concerned about political careers as well as winning the next election. The 'Why?' is not answered by health care: the 'Why?' is answered by what the important issues are going to be in the next election and the most important issue is the economy. If you do not believe me ask yourself how people would vote if given the choice of a private health care system or a five per cent reduction in the mortgage rate. The economy is an important electoral factor from which lots of other changes flow. So the 'Why?' is about building an economic platform, building an economic dynamic that can help win the next election. The 'What?' is to increase private investment, to increase the sale of assets that is boosting the economy now; and 'How?' is to get public sector services ready for privatization.

I am not asking you to answer the question 'Which of these two views is real?' All I am asking you to admit is that both of those views exist. If you do not believe me, ask yourself why the ambulance dispute went on so long. Was it about better health care, or was it about the economy? And if you still do not believe me, let me tell you about changes that are happening elsewhere.

The Civil Service—although we like to think that the Health Service is the centre for all progressive, dynamic change—is going through a period of change which makes changes in the Health Service look minuscule. The entire Civil Service is being reorganized into agencies on contract to central policy units. These agencies are contract agencies which might in future be privatized, but are now being being set up as public benefit corporations on contract to their policy units. This is not just happening in places like Vehicle Licensing but is also happening in places like the Department of Social Security, which is becoming an agency during the next 12 months.

The organization that I work with—the Office for Public Management—looks at changes in public management generally. The kinds of changes that are occurring around the construction of agencies are very interesting, progressive to some extent, and we have been trying to explore why this is happening. Recently we have met with people in some of the Conservative Party think-tanks about why it is that they are doing so much to improve public management. Why it is that management is really the focus of what they are doing. In the middle of our questioning, we were interrupted to say, 'Let us get this absolutely clear: this is not "Why?" management; this is about how to bust the public sector unions and about how to cut public expenditure. In order to do that you need strong tools, and our tool is management.'

Now, I am not picking sides: I am saying that either Kenneth Clarke or Major Lawson may well be right. Those of us who believe this is all about getting a better deal for us may be right, but those who believe that this is about bigger things are probably also right. The end result is that there isn't a commonly held answer to why this is all happening and that is resulting in confusion. People do not know why they are doing what they are doing and they are responding in two ways: they are responding through fear, and they are responding through flattery.

As I said earlier, the responsibility of those who are being flattered is to tell people what they want to hear. What the people in Whitehall want to hear is that the White Paper is working, so when we come back from our US visits we talk about the enterprise culture, about innovation, about doctors and management, and about how it can all work. The most flattered people in the group, the people who are carrying this message most strongly I think, are Health Service managers. There is a view that the White Paper is about better management, about business plans, about contracts, and about Resource Management Initiative. Well, aside from the lessons that we see in the Civil Service, I think that we should begin to focus on the fact that what is actually happening as a result of this flattery is that management is becoming reified—management is becoming important in its own right. But management is not a product nor is it a value. It is not an idea that results from the process. It is a method. It is simply a means, and yet the flatterers and those being flattered are being caught in the means. They are being caught up in the fact that they are in there to do the 'What?' and the 'How?' and not to answer the 'Why?'. This is not the case with all Health Service managers: there are some who are much more interested in health outcomes than in hospital contracts—some who you will hear from today—and those managers are beginning to form an alternative force.

The second response is that of fear. Now, remember that the response of fear is not to tell people what they do not want to hear. What they do not want to hear is that the health of the population is not about purchaser/providers. It is about health enhancement, about health maintenance, and about a healthy social and economic environment. But you do not say that. You do not come back from the States and say, 'Yes, well there may be enterprise and initiative but there are Visa-carded admissions, there are 35 million people who do not have health care, and teaching hospitals are going bankrupt.' Instead, you keep your head down, you play the fear game and do not say anything that is going to disturb. The people who are most guilty of this, in my view, are people in Community Medicine—I won't call them people in Public Health. Community Medicine over the last year has rediscovered epidemiology. Epidemiology has become important in its own right. 'Factor analysis' and 'causal modelling', even 'medical audit', have become the key words. But once again epidemiology is not a product, it is not a value, it is not even a theory or an idea—it is simply a means. Not everybody in Community Medicine is fearful. Once again, there are people who are much more interested in health programmes than in diagnostic-related groups. They too are beginning to form a small alternative force.

What do we do, as we go through the first birthday of the working paper, to deal with fear and flattery—the two new emotions around the White Paper? I think three things.

One is to focus on health results. How many of us have actually spent time asking ourselves or our organizations what we expect the outcomes of all of this to be. I work with one organization—you will also hear from Alasdair Liddell this afternoon—whose regional executive is actually making time as an executive with clinicians to begin to consider the questions: 'What is health? What are we here for?' How many of us have spent time focusing our efforts, our organizations, on health outcomes? I think the first thing we must do is begin to get the health argument back on the agenda. This is not about business plans, it is not about contracts; it is about health.

Secondly, I think we must begin to focus on assuring the health of the population, and this means focusing on the role of districts. I think we can let the Department and management development centres deal with business plans and hospital contracts, but we have to seize the initiative and define a new, assuring role for the District Health Authorities. For managers, the important role in this is defining a new type of accountability. It is not about money—it is about access, it is about equity, and it is even about democracy. For public health there is a big role here too, and it is helping to define the new product. It is not about meeting patterns of cardiovascular disease—it is about stress, occupational patterns, local education, and the economy. We need new Directors of Public Health who understand that 'public' is just as important as 'health' in their titles.

Thirdly and finally, I think we have to stop pretending to be either flattered or fearful. Certainly, we have to discuss the answers to 'What?' and 'How?', but we also have to provide the answers to 'Why?'. Answering the question 'Why?' is a unique role of leadership and I think we have to become the leaders. Kenneth Clarke and Major Lawson, Robin Cook and John Smith are not going to provide the answers to 'Why?' in a way which talks about health outcome. The agenda for them is different and bigger. The leadership in answering 'Why?' has to come from managers and people in public health, the only people in whose hands the Health Service can be safe. So I hope that as we approach a second birthday, the little forces that are beginning to grow will do away with fear and flattery, and will begin to form a forceful, fearless leadership that begins to put health back on the agenda.

I hope that today we can have a good meeting, that we can learn a lot, and that we can emerge from all of this a bit less flattered and a lot less fearful than we were when we began.

Chairman: Thank you very much indeed Dr Parston. You took us on a very interesting voyage across a very wide territory, and as far as I was concerned I was very happy where you ended up. I can say that I think if anyone was sleepy when they arrived here, I doubt if there is anyone half asleep now.

Session 1: Information for health

SIR DONALD ACHESON—Chairman

3

Needs assessment

DR DEIRDRE CUNNINGHAM

Today I am talking in the context of being the Director of Public Health of a large inner London district, as well as the Chairman, until last Monday, of a consortium of districts and academic departments who have joined together to work on assessment of needs. I can only skim the surface of needs so I am not going to touch on all aspects of this vast topic.

Needs assessment is not new. It has been bread and butter work for public health physicians and many other specialties for decades. 'Need' has become a jargon word although there are a range of different interpretations. It might therefore be helpful to clarify this by looking at some definitions.

I have gone to the earliest English dictionary to see what Samuel Johnson in 1755 thought of 'need' (Table 1). What I found was interesting: first of all he comes across a biblical definition of 'need', but secondly 'want' and 'need' were then apparently almost synonymous. I think we could remember this today: that what I want is not necessarily what somebody else feels I need.

Table 1. Samuel Johnson's definition of 'need' (*A dictionary of the English language*, 1755)

Need

1. Exigency; pressing difficulty; necessity.
2. Want; distressful poverty.
3. Want; lack of anything for use.
   'The whole need not a physician, but the sick'
   Matt. ix.12.

How has 'need' been defined in health care settings? I am sure we all know many definitions: Matthew, Bradshaw's taxonomy, Glass, etc. One member of my Department was trying to define 'need' and felt he could do an MD on this, taking two years. We agreed that we didn't have that much time, so we looked at how other people had defined 'needs'.

Knox, in his *Epidemiology and health care planning* published in 1979, actually used the definition by Donobedian: 'Some disturbance in health and well-being which requires medical services'. We might actually say 'health care services' rather than 'medical services'. Knox has some observations in his book about feeding needs into the planning cycle, and what he points out is that health care planners require estimates of continued 'need', not just point prevalence. Whatever you are planning actually comes on stream in a year or two hence, and therefore you require 'need' to be updated: group rather than individual needs, quantitative as well as qualitative. He also pointed out the very important point that 'need' is always a perception. Whose perception?

'Needs' cannot only be defined by professionals. 'Need' and 'want' are not always synonymous, as McCarthy discussed in *Epidemiology and policies for health planning* and published in 1982. McCarthy also pointed out that 'need' is not easy to define. You can actually descriptively record professionally identified 'need' in a survey, although the individual may not wish to receive care or treatment for that 'need'. Certainly in Parkside we have very carefully assessed the need for a cervical screening programme, we have implemented it, and have evaluated it over two years. It is quite apparent that a large proportion of the women in our district do not actually want it. We similarly know that many women do not want high-tech deliveries; they want their babies to be delivered at home. But *we* feel that they ought to be delivered in hospitals. Similarly for anti-smoking messages: respiratory and cardiovascular disease would actually be reduced if we stopped people smoking. But do people want to hear these messages and stop smoking?

Many analogies exist relating to 'needs' and all of them highlight one important point: 'whatever you do, however many needs you meet, there is always the aspect of unmet need'. Again, McCarthy highlighted three of these analogies:

one is Greg Parston's 'onion concept' and there is Last and Hannay's 'iceberg concept'; Abel-Smith introduced the concept of 'cost' which we cannot ignore.

Some form of needs assessment has been used in all health care delivery systems in either a systematic or on an *ad hoc* basis. The USA and Canada are good examples. They vary in their level of sophistication and applicability to this country, so I am not going to go over all the models of needs assessment that I have come across. One or two are worth scrutinizing. The one I am going to suggest which could be a useful model, and might well be adopted here, is that of the US Preventive Services Task Force. This Task Force followed an earlier Canadian one, and its findings were published late in 1989. As such, the document is not yet widely available in the UK.

A group of eminent physicians and other health professionals met 14 times over four years from 1984 to 1988, to assess the published evidence and make recommendations on 169 preventive interventions. For each intervention a recommendation was made ranging from (a)—there is good evidence to support the recommendation that the condition be specifically considered in a periodic health examination—to (e)—there is good evidence that it should be excluded from consideration (Table 2). The quality of the evidence was graded from I to III: I was assigned when evidence had been obtained from at least one properly designed, randomized control trial and III when evidence was still based on the opinions of respected authorities (Table 3).

Thus, for HIV infection, when they looked at HIV antibody testing the quality of the evidence was assessed as a III; i.e. still at the opinion stage. Their recommendation for people from identified risk groups was (b): there was fair evidence that HIV antibody testing should be performed, which included pregnant women, whilst poor evidence existed for individuals not at risk (c). For common childhood infections, such as diphtheria, tetanus, whooping cough, mumps, and rubella, the intervention was vaccination, the quality of the evidence was graded as I, and the recommendation was (a), appropriate for everybody.

Table 2: Strength of recommendations according to the US Preventive Services Task Force, 1989

(a) There is good evidence to support the recommendation that the condition be specifically considered in a periodic health examination.
(b) There is fair evidence to support the recommendation that the condition be specifically considered in a periodic health examination.
(c) There is poor evidence regarding the inclusion of the condition in a periodic health examination, but recommendations may be made on other grounds.
(d) There is fair evidence to support the recommendation that the condition be excluded from consideration in a periodic health examination.
(e) There is good evidence to support the recommendation that the condition be excluded from consideration in a periodic health examination.

Table 3: Quality of evidence according to the US Preventive Services Task Force, 1989

I. Evidence obtained from at least one properly-designed, randomized controlled trial.
II-1. Evidence obtained from well-designed controlled trials without randomization.
II-2. Evidence obtained from well-designed cohort or case-control analytic studies, preferably from more than one centre or research group.
II-3. Evidence obtained from multiple time series with or without the intervention. Dramatic results in uncontrolled experiments (such as the results of the introduction of penicillin treatment in the 1940s) could also be regarded as this type of evidence.
III. Opinions of respected authorities, based on clinical experience, descriptive studies, or reports of expert committees.

I feel the American publication will be immensely useful for both districts and the medical and nursing colleges in developing preventive services. The team actually said that the process of developing these recommendations was almost as important for medical policy as the actual outcome, and maintained that this method could be transferred to treatment.

When the White Paper came out, what data did we have to draw on to assess needs and implement the recommendations? I am sure you all know these: we had a lot of mortality data, which included crude, standardized, cause-specific and occupation-specific mortality data. Additional to small area mortality data we have had avoidable deaths packages with aggregated mortality data over a few years. These indicate sentinel events which are avoidable and should not happen, and which might be used as indicators of potential bad practice. We have had morbidity measures, which are notoriously incomplete. Infectious disease notification may be improved when the legislation is reviewed but all these proxy measures could be better. There may also be more local information available collected in an *ad hoc* way. These *ad hoc* measures that we are familiar with include prevalence or incidence studies. Some people are doing health status surveys. Numerous other epidemiological methods exist. Two methods can be viewed as possible, useful, practical, and pragmatic models; both already existed when the White Paper came out. These could form a basis of the type of model the district might like to use in their needs assessment.

The first is the Forrest Report—which you may not have thought of as a form of needs assessment (Fig. 1). This formal assessment of needs for the given target population enables districts or screening centres to take a target population, apply formulae for percentages who attend and percentages who wish treatment, and to derive total screening attendances, total referrals for assessment, and total referrals for biopsy and breast cancers detected. Now, if we developed assessments of needs in this standardized format—one page with boxes that districts could fill in according to an agreed formula—it would be possible to look at service requirements. This would include screening service requirements, assessment and biopsy requirements, as well as the medical manpower required to perform them. This could then be used to assess the total numbers of mastectomies or lumpectomies and other services that a district might wish to purchase.

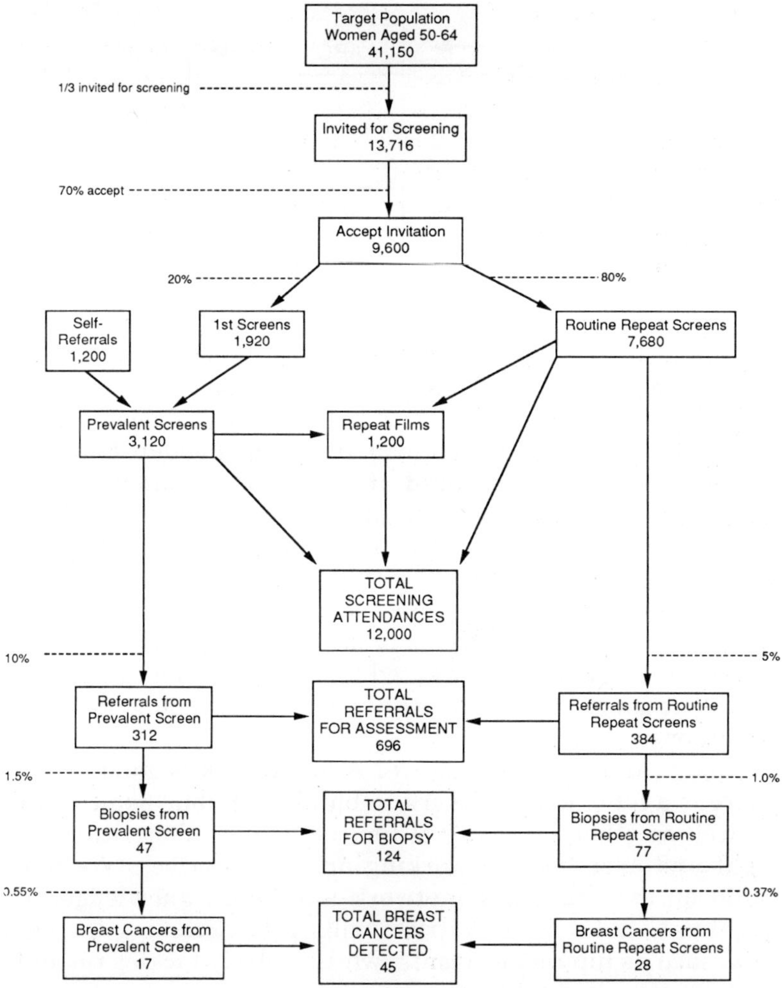

Fig. 1. Estimated annual number of women undergoing different stages of the screening process in an established programme in a population of 471000 served by the basic screening unit (4th and subsequent years). (DHSS Breast Cancer Screening, 1986.)

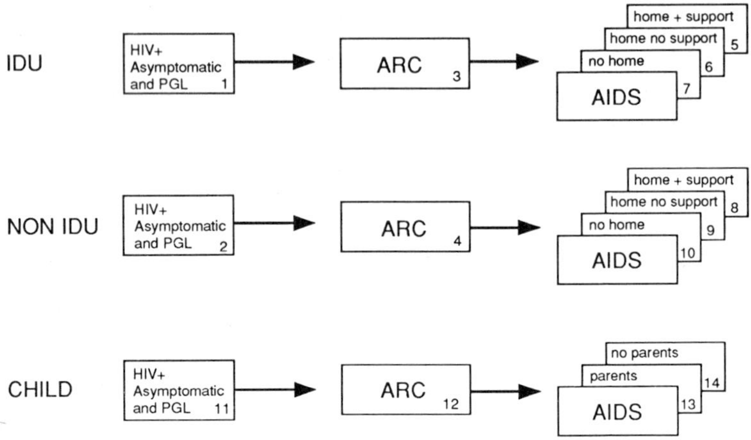

Fig. 2. Categories of patients with HIV infection (according to Rosenhead 1989).

Similarly, the Rosenhead Model (Fig. 2) is a model for care for people with HIV infection, asymptomatic or symptomatic, commissioned by Parkside Health Authority and developed by Professor Jonathan Rosenhead from the London School of Economics. He has produced an interactive computer model which you can interrogate to identify the needs for care for such patients. He has divided HIV patients into three categories: injecting drug-user (IDU), non-drug-user, or child. He has divided them into disease stages as well as existing home and support conditions and identified packages of care which were required and wanted for each condition. We feel we could transfer this model to what we are doing for other conditions.

One year on—where are we? A lot of work is going on and there is a lot of existing work to build on. Public health skills as well as other skills are of limited supply. Time-scales are tight and everybody is working around the clock. We must build on existing work, network and share knowledge. My nightmare is that 190 districts will all be assessing the easy bits, such as hip replacements, whilst nobody tackles the difficult issues like mental health care. The Faculty of Public Health Medicine has already recognized this and has agreed to try to disseminate around the country examples of existing good practice. Examples of current work include the third annual health report from Central Birmingham Health Authority. This has been turned over to look at assessment of needs and feeding them into the contracting processes, called *Buying better health: risk and opportunity or crisis*.

There are currently many consortia and I am aware that many of these are pooling their skills all round the country. I am going to describe the activities of one consortium for assessment of needs which we have set up in North East and North West Thames Districts. It involves five district public health departments: Barnet, Bloomsbury, Hampstead, Islington, and Parkside—one academic public health department, that of St. Mary's Hospital Medical School, and one GP research unit largely concerned with the elderly, the Helen Hamlyn Research Unit. We are working to two time-scales: one is rapid, developing pragmatic models for assessing need, bearing in mind the need for quality, to produce base-lines for annual health reports in October 1990 and to be used by planners and purchasers before then. The other will obviously require more detailed work on a longer time-scale producing work which we hope might be generalizable. Each project has a project leader and each district or department is taking on at least one if not more projects. We have decided to take a disease-based approach to this. Questions to be answered by every project leader include: (i) What databases or information are available? (ii) What are the data requirements? (iii) What are the current levels of unmet, met, and overmet need? (iv) What treatment or services are applicable to the topic? (v) Are the outcomes of these acceptable, unacceptable, or effective? (vi) At what threshold should individuals be accepted into these services? (vii) What methods are available for internal or external monitoring? Do acceptable criteria for use in audit exist? (viii) What methods are available for prioritizing? If we cannot actually afford to provide all levels of care, what are the most crucial issues?

Our initial projects include major health issues in terms of mortality, morbidity, and health service use. They are posing some problems. The first issue we tackled in Parkside was ischaemic heart disease. We are also involved with stroke, diabetes, pregnancy, and childbirth. We feel these are all crunch issues for the first year of contracting. Other conditions have a substantial elective surgery component, such as hip disease, and could equally apply to cataracts or other operations, and there is a third category of those conditions with a recognized and funded screening component, such as breast disease. We have not yet tackled conditions significantly involving other authorities and we have not cracked the hard ones, like mental illness.

We started off assessing the needs of special groups separately. We have now decided that for the elderly, homeless, people from ethnic minorities, and other groups which might require special attention, we are not actually going to assess their needs separately and independently. Rather, we are using a matrix enabling our disease-based assessment of needs to be broken down by demographic and social groups as well as by service or service delivery component to make it useful for planning. So we will have a matrix with numbers and information in the boxes which we can produce in any form that the purchasers require.

We have developed a schematic representation of our needs assessment model (Fig. 3), which allows us to proceed from identifying important conditions which are amenable to medical care. We assume we are identifying contemporary needs for medical or health care. One can go round the circle to estimate the percentage of people who are going to take up treatment and one can therefore calculate the quantity you will need to purchase. The problem is that we are trying to identify those conditions amenable to medical or health care interventions and we are rather stuck on the information available on their effectiveness. We have assumed that those interventions of unknown efficacy should be given the benefit of the doubt until we have evidence to the contrary. I ultimately see no sensible way to get this without actually feeding in the results of audit into the assessment of needs process. Perhaps here also the Royal Colleges might wish to actually undertake assessments of the effectiveness of medical interventions.

One year on—is more theory required? I think probably not. We know a lot about needs. I always remember a conference in Paddington and North Kensington where one of the participants said, 'We get fed up with people asking us what we need if they are not prepared to do anything about it.'

This illustrates that it is all very well identifying needs; how are we going to get decisions made on the basis of them? Logically, and this may be unpalatable, the implication is that we may be closing services which we cannot demonstrate are

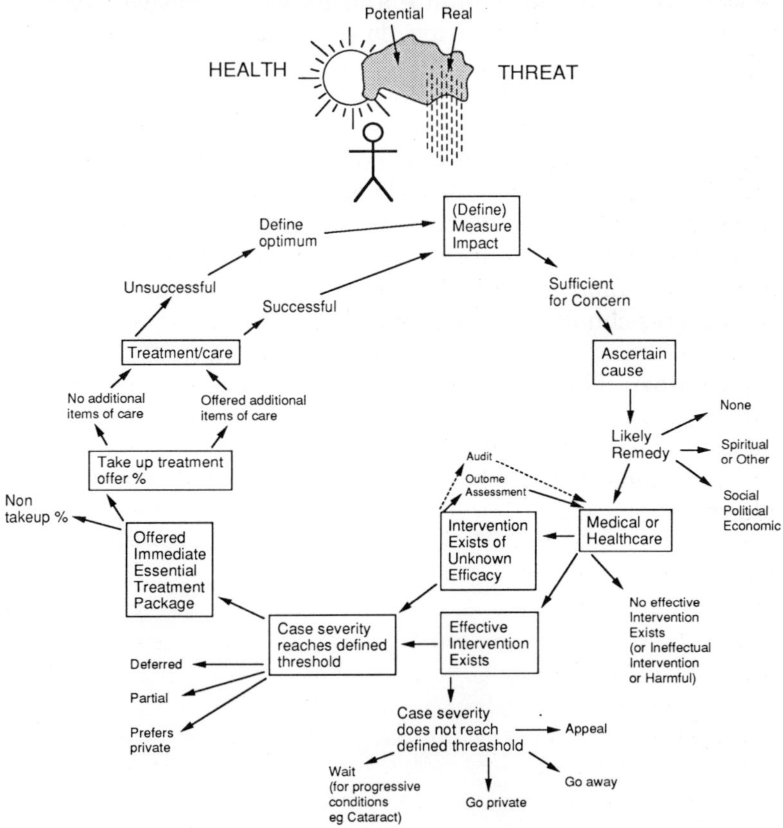

Fig. 3. Schematic representation of a needs assessment model.

needed. This is in order to free up resources, including people, for those that we can demonstrate are needed. The NHS and other organizations are always very good at adding things on, but not very good at taking things off. We are not flexible.

Finally, a few maxims on needs assessment. We must be realistic—certainly with ischaemic heart disease we do not reckon we can get much beyond calculating the status quo of health care received and the use and demand in the first year for that condition. We may not even manage that. We must build on work already undertaken here, in the USA, and elsewhere. We must disseminate and network; however bad our information is, we can always do something. I am going to end with a quote which illustrates that 'needs' is a tool rather an end in itself. According to Russell in 1989: 'Ultimately the services included in a National Health Plan depend on the resources available, on alternatives for the use of those resources, and on people's judgement about the value of the alternatives. Cost effectiveness evaluations on needs assessment make the alternatives clearer and can help ensure that our choices more truly reflect what we care about'; 'we' being both professionals and the public.

Chairman: Thank you very much, Deirdre, for covering so much ground and I feel sure your comment that there might be a role for Royal Colleges in determining the effectiveness of interventions has not been lost on this audience and in this place.

4

Medical audit

PROFESSOR SIR RAYMOND HOFFENBERG

The term 'medical audit' is used in so many different senses and in so many different ways that I am not going to attempt a definition. There is a very good definition in the Working Paper No. 6 of the White Paper, which I would commend to you. Classically, as we know, three elements in service provision are recognized: those of structure, process, and outcome. The point I wish to make is that all three are important and they are wholly interdependent. From a managerial point of view, I think it correct that the emphasis should be on the optimum use of resources or value for money. In order to achieve this, it is necessary to analyse structure and to know what resources are available. It is also necessary to analyse the process of how these resources are being used. But the exercise would be sterile—and I suggest might even be harmful to the Health Service—if managers concentrated entirely on maximizing the use of resources and failed to take account of outcome. From the opposite point of view, the clinician's point of view, the essence of medical care is its outcome or the result of intervention. Inevitably, this will depend on structure and process. The purpose of studying outcome must always be to try to improve structure and process; to modify them in order to achieve a better outcome. Medical audit would indeed be a waste of time and effort if it were not to lead to improvements in health care.

One of the problems is that the measurement of outcome is not easy. It has to take account of inherent variations between individuals, within and between communities and populations. Some elements of outcome, however, are readily quantifiable and death is the obvious one. You can measure length of stay in hospital or the time taken for full recovery, for instance to return to work. Even these apparently straightforward indices need careful appraisal. They depend to a large extent on the nature of the patients to whom they are being applied. An excellent unit might have the highest mortality rates or the longest stay in hospital simply because complex and advanced patients are being referred to it in recognition of its excellence.

In general, I think surgery lends itself more readily to outcome analysis than medicine. A large part of surgery is concerned with the management of a relatively acute episode or an elective operation in an individual who is or was otherwise quite well, someone who could be expected to return to a full, normal, and active life. Surgical procedures—for instance a cholecystectomy or hernia repair—are relatively standardized. They make it easier therefore to interpret the outcome and also to compare the results from one surgeon to another, or from one institution to another. Length of stay in hospital, readmissions, time to return to work—all of these have some relationship to the quality of surgical care. Complications such as bleeding or infection are well defined and usually easily recognized and measurable.

Audit of medical processes is less easy. Medical patients often have chronic and complex problems, investigations and treatments are less standardized and criteria of outcome less precise. The end points are less easily identified, apart from death. Death has formed the basis of very informative studies, such as the report that came from the Royal College of Physicians on deaths under the age of 50, Lunn and Mushins' reported deaths associated with anaesthesia, or that aspect of the Confidential Enquiry on Peri-Operative Deaths (CEPOD) Report from the Royal College of Surgeons. Problems are encountered in medical situations when less precise criteria are used. We see this, for instance, in some studies of recurrent myocardial infarction which are based on clinical or ECG criteria. We see it where observer interpretation is important, for instance in pathological or scan appearances. It is not easy to get good comparative data for the management of chronic diseases, like rheumatoid arthritis, or patients who have had strokes, because the problem here becomes the assessment of that less tangible and less easily measured entity 'quality of life'. That, however, is too big a problem for me to try to tackle now.

One of the most striking aspects of the CEPOD Report of the College of Surgeons was the suggestion that as many as 20 per cent of all deaths were attributable to avoidable surgical or anaesthetic factors. This raises the awkward question of individual medical accountability and the assessment of individual competence. In her book, *Rules, roles and relations*, Dorothy Emmett makes the point that a profession carries with it the notion of a standard of performance and that it has a fiduciary trust to maintain standards. These are partly standards of competence or technical ability, but they are also joined with professional integrity. The question we have to ask is: 'How do we, as medical professionals, judge the competence and integrity of our colleagues?' Without making any objective analysis, it is fair to say that we usually have a pretty shrewd idea of the quality of care offered by other doctors. We recognize good practitioners and we recognize bad practitioners. General practitioners tend to refer their patents to consultants who they recognize provide high-quality medical care. Consultants know which of their colleagues to call in when they or their families need attention. We have recognized within the profession that medicine is practised across a wide range of standards—some are good, some excellent, and some regrettably are bad. If some standards are unacceptably bad for us or our families, why should they be tolerated for our patients? Do we not have a duty, Dorothy Emmett's fiduciary trust, to ensure that everyone receives medical care of a standard that we would accept for our own? This can only be done if we establish criteria for good medical practice and set up procedures for its appraisal. In other words, if we set up an intraprofessional system of audit.

In this regard I would like just to mention a system which we introduced in the professorial unit in Birmingham more than 12 years ago. At a regular weekly meeting, we scrutinized the case notes and discussed the management of individual patients by individual doctors. This was done in the presence of consultants, junior staff and medical students. A modified form of this scheme has been recommended in the Royal College of Physicians' Report on Medical Audit which was published at the beginning of 1989. The Joint Committee for Higher Medical Training has adopted the recommendations of the College and approval of training posts may now be withheld or withdrawn if satisfactory audit procedures are not in place. I think that is quite a big step forward.

In considering the management of individual medical problems, differences of opinion are bound to arise. The ensuing debate that takes place at these meetings often leads to literature reviews, occasionally to fresh research, in an endeavour to find the truth. In other words, the audit meetings have a very strong educational value as well. There will of course always be uncertainties and variations in practice and it should not be our aim to abolish these. We should not be trying to get all doctors to conform to standard clinical practices according to established algorithms. We do, however, need to know whether extremes or marked departures from standard clinical behaviour are justified or acceptable. Government is not unaware of these variations in medical practice throughout the country, and in the introduction to the White Paper one finds statements such as these: 'In 1986/87 the average cost of treating acute hospital in-patients varied by as much as 50 per cent between different health authorities, even after allowing for the complexity and mix of cases treated.' Or, 'A patient who waited several years for an operation in one place may get that same operation within a few weeks in another.' Or, 'In some places drug costs are nearly twenty times as high per head of population as in others.' Or, 'There is a twenty-fold variation in the rate at which GPs refer patients to hospitals.' These findings are unquestionably true, they come from a source that one could not possibly question, and they require an explanation. They must not simply be interpreted as evidence of inefficiency or wastefulness by those places that spend more, have the lowest patient throughput or longest waiting lists. There could easily be other explanations.

Government spokesmen talk of introducing systems like the Diagnosis Related Group (DRG) which will tend to standardize the clinical management of certain conditions. In the United States, as we know, almost 500 sets of DRG guidelines are now in use and they form the basis of third-party payments. This is a rather rigid system of medical care in which clinicians are required to justify deviations from the norm. If, for instance, you are allowed four days of hospital admission for a hernia operation, on the morning of day five, if your patient is still there, you get a telephone call from the financing department of the hospital saying, 'Why is your patient still here?' This now happens widely and regularly.

It appears that DRGs are causing increasing dissatisfaction in the US. They are not cheap. In the first year of their introduction the costs of medical care went up by roughly 8·5 per cent against an anticipated 3·5 per cent and, as we all know, costs in America are continuing to rise. It must also be said that in this country we have no real idea at present of how to determine optimal DRG practices or how to cost them. I guess it will take years before we assemble rational and acceptable figures.

As an aside, I heard a Regional Health Authority manager earlier this week suggesting that audit and costing of clinical teaching would now be necessary. He went on to say that the content, duration, and quality of teaching should all be assessed in financial terms. As an ex-medical academic, I would love to know the basis for judging these matters which certainly academic medicine cannot do.

In recent years, Government has introduced clinical performance indicators (PIs) and other measures of hospital activity. PIs, Sir Kenneth Stowe said at their time of their introduction, essentially comprise rankings of all the 192 districts in the English Health Service in competitive order of performance against certain indicators. McGuire has pointed out that in the United Kingdom they are not wholly concerned with measuring improvements in health care, nor are they solely concerned with variations in medical practice. He said rather, that they are 'measures of throughput and resources introduced to tighten the monitoring and control of the NHS in order to contain expenditure'.

Clinical PIs must not be used as a device to drive expenditure down to the lowest level or to force units to handle more patients, perform more operations, or reduce hospital stay—not at least without careful assessment of the clinical consequences. If this is their purpose we will end up practising what the Americans call 'revolving door medicine' as a result of which one senator said, 'patients are being discharged quicker and sicker'. Variations in rates and costs of treatment are known to persist in widely divergent medical systems, in the US as well as in this country. They are more readily explained by uncertainties in medical practice than by inefficiency. This is not to say that our system is devoid of waste or inefficiency in medical practice. Where it does exist we must find and eliminate it. I suspect that our demands for more money for the Health Service would carry more weight if we did so.

Our main problem is the paucity of information on which to base judgements about better practice. As Dr Cunningham mentioned earlier, there is still too little known about outcome. Again, in this College, our research unit, which was established some 10 or 12 years ago, has been modified completely. We have a new director and its objective now is to set up outcome studies that we hope will eventually lead to clearer guidelines for the basis of medical treatment.

To do this we will require substantial Government investment. One has to be prepared to spend a lot of money on large-scale trials and detailed, well thought-out studies of outcome. It is going to demand much clinician time, and this, I am afraid, will require expansion of medical staff numbers, particularly at the consultant level. It is quite unrealistic to expect clinicians to find time for these activities in addition to everything else that they are now being asked to do.

In closing, I would just like to say that I have given some sound professional reasons for supporting the introduction of medical audit, to improve standards of care, to raise awareness of costs, to eliminate waste and inefficiency, and, I believe, to institute a valuable educational tool. I think there is a less professional reason for introducing audit by doctors. That is, if doctors themselves do not do it somebody else will, and I suspect it will not be half as good.

Chairman: Thank you very much for that very thoughtful summary of so many of the issues relating to audit.

5

Resource management

DR JOHN MITCHELL

The Government has set a very ambitious timetable for the implementation of the resource management initiative. We now have the six original pilot sites which have been joined by 20 others and another 30 will come on stream for the introduction of resource management over the course of the next year. The Government's stated aim is that all 260 acute hospitals in the country will have resource management implemented by 1992. As health authorities, hospitals, and the Department invest ever increasing time, energy, money, and resources, I think it is essential that we consider who is trying to achieve what by this initiative.

To try and answer this question, I would like to make three major points. First, that resource management is primarily about means and not ends. Second, that resource management requires continual and profound organizational change; and third—perhaps the most important—that local managers and their professional colleagues have an essential and important role and responsibility in leading their hospitals and units to provide quality care outcomes.

The thinking that resource management is an end in itself comes from a number of sources. Kenneth Clarke, in his introduction to the Resource Management Initiative Information Pack, pointed out, 'the importance of resource management is difficult to overstate, particularly with new and more reliable information on activity and cost'. He then went on to link resource management to self-governing hospitals and making them work.

David Willetts, Director of the Centre of Policy Studies and the prospective Conservative parliamentary candidate for Havant, went one step further when he said, 'It is also needs management arrangement which will give doctors and nurses power and responsibility to act on that information.' These views I think have been strengthened by the way the initiative is being financially driven from the centre. The objectives appear straightforward. To introduce an information system and appoint clinical directors as early as possible while concurrently preparing a number of hospitals for self-governance. Essentially the Government wishes to demonstrate its policies for acute services are well-intentioned and needs examples of good-quality health care to be operative by the time the next election comes round.

Obviously, I agree that professionals—particularly doctors—should be intimately involved in managing hospitals, and that we need accurate and timely information. If, however, these are the only aspects conceived as being important when implementing resource management then I have no confidence that it will significantly improve the quality of clinical services for a number of reasons.

The first is that it fails to address one of the major managerial challenges in the NHS: the need to reconcile the tension between guidance and delivery management. Between those people who are trying to steer their organizations, hospitals, or authorities, through the difficult political, financial, and policy environment and those who are primarily concerned with delivering day-to-day health care, which includes professionals who are trying to meet the needs of individual people. Reconciling this tension is a major managerial challenge which resource management in its restricted form will not be able to address.

The second is that it is exceedingly difficult to install appropriate information systems that can cope with the complexities of case-mix, DRGs, coding, nursing, costs, audit, and so on. Unless the organization itself has a clear understanding and idea of what it is trying to do, and there is clear agreement in the organization about what its role is, the chance of wasting significant financial resources is high.

Thirdly, if one appoints clinical directors, who are likely to be doctors, to organizations which have no clearly defined purpose and role, they will at best become efficient pragmatists and at worse disillusioned antagonists in the process of managing health care. It is likely therefore that this could result in more division than we have at the present time.

The final point is epitomized by a recent experience. We have recently had 20 clinical directors working at the King's Fund College and we asked them to provide answers to the question: 'What do other doctors think resource management is?' This resulted in a list of many views including: 'cost containment', 'a straight jacket', 'fashionable jargon', 'limitation of clinical freedom', and 'another unnecessary change'. The list is uniformly negative. We went on to ask them what they thought managers saw in resource management. The list is equally depressing: 'controlling doctors', 'passing the buck to clinicians', 'clinical control', and so on. There are one or two more positive ones, but generally their views about this were equally negative. I should add that when we asked a group of managers the same questions, they would come out with the same stereotypical views.

I think these responses illustrate just how dislocated many hospital organizations are. These feelings of distrust are so prevalent that I would argue that the provision of information systems or the appointment of some clinical directors themselves, will not significantly improve the outcome of clinical services.

This brings me on to the second major theme which I wish to discuss, namely organizational change. It seems to me that, if resource management is going to improve the quality of service, each hospital will need to undergo profound and continual change. To illustrate what I mean, I would like to refer to some work that Otto Brodrick and his colleagues did for the Canadian Auditor General and described by Dye in *Attributes of well-performing organizations : study by the Office of the Auditor General, Canada* in 1988. They looked at eight selected 'well-performing' public sector organizations in Canada and described their important common organizational characteristics.

The first conclusion that they drew was that these public 'bureaucracies' were thinking and behaving more like public 'enterprises': they had moved from being organizations which were characterized by red tape and unresponsiveness to ones that were innovative, responsive, and productive. There had been a shift in the organizational culture.

They identified four major attributes that were common to these organizations, which will not come as any surprise to you: an emphasis on people, the concept of participative or democratic leadership, innovative work styles, and strong client orientation. I would like to look at those individual features in a little more detail to provide some understanding of what they were talking about.

1. *An emphasis on people*: in the well-performing organization there was a strong belief in people to act, make judgements, and produce high performance. People were preoccupied with success, risk-taking was encouraged, and new issues were seen as a challenge. In the poor-performance organization, the emphasis was on systems and procedures which constrain individual performance, people were likely to be preoccupied with failure, risk-taking was discouraged, and new issues were seen as a problem.
2. *Participative leadership*: the well-performing organizations had a clear definition of the goals and purpose which were articulated to the organization. Commitment to the organization was fostered continually; hearing and listening were commonplace and part of the culture. Where individual accountability was clear, hierarchy and boundaries were not regarded as important. Conversely, in poor-performance organizations, goals are unclear and purpose indefinable; being uncommitted is seen as normal. Hierarchies were used and formal levels imposed and considered to be important, to create a closed communication style.
3. *Innovative workstyle*: well-performing organizations learnt to do things differently persistently; they had self-controlled open feedback and evaluation systems. They were self-reliant in problem-solving capabilities and reviewed and consulted routinely as well as celebrating their successes. Conversely, in poor-

performance organizations learning might go on for individuals but the organization itself did not benefit. There were rigid external control and feedback systems and such organizations mainly reacted and responded to external demands and control. They characteristically consulted formally but seldom reviewed progress or celebrated success.

4. *Strong client orientation*: in well-performing organizations great satisfaction was gained from serving their clients. There was a strong interaction and relationship between the clients and the organization and a welcoming of client feedback. Whereas, in the poor-performance organization the bureaucracy was served and not the client. The relationship between the client and the organization tended to be weak, there was often a defensiveness about what the client thought, and the views of the clients were likely to be ignored.

It seems to me that while individuals or even individual departments might have features that are well-performing, hospitals themselves very seldom perform in that sort of way globally. I would suggest that what we are talking about is the need for significant organizational change in trying to shift the organizations to behave like those Canadian well-performing organizations and adopt some of their characteristics.

Something that is terribly important as part of the adaptation is the concept of values. Brodrick defined it as 'a mind set which seeks optimum performance and achieves agreed values despite changing conditions'. A sense that the whole time people are looking to do things better, that they use an explicit set of values to work from despite an overall environment which is continually changing. Whether through White Papers, economic availability, or whatever, they have to cope continually with these changes.

A couple of other points about these well-performing organizations are worth noting. Good information systems were not necessarily characteristic of them. Our own obsession with information at the moment therefore urgently needs to be readdressed in this context. They further emphasize the importance of non-hierarchical organizations and, therefore, a structural solution of putting doctors in a position of accountability as clinical directors may not necessarily result in the desired objectives.

I have a colleague who talks about resource management as though it were a stool: the three legs of the stool are represented by three features of information systems, structures/clinical directorships, and organizational change. I think this analogy nicely points out that unless you have these three components the stool will fall over and resource management will not work. I have an alternative model which is that of an ocean-going trimaran: the central hull, the mast, the rigging, and the steering represent the organization, its culture, and the change required; the two additional hulls on either side represent the clinical director structure and the information systems respectively. The latter two will clearly improve the performance and add more potential, but unless you have the central component the initiative is meaningless. I would argue the importance of understanding how we have to change the organizations in which we work if we want to start delivering quality services at the end of the day.

My third major point concerns local managers and professionals. They have a major responsibility to provide leadership and vision. This to ensure that hospitals and other units have the capacity and ability to respond to and provide for the health needs of their local communities. They have to ask themselves three critical questions. First, is there any agreement and understanding within the organization of what the hospital is trying to do? Second, is it producing quality services uniformly? And third, does the hospital have the appropriate organizational characteristics which will enable it to deliver a quality product? We need to develop a clear sense of honesty and openness about what is really going on. Certainly, there are good things, innovative ideas, satisfied patients, caring and concerned staff; but are our overall services really excellent?

The time for defending the indefensible has passed. If we do not start providing services which serve the user, ensuring choice and enabling self-determination, services which are increasingly more skilful and appropriate to the needs of the individual and the population, then we are threatening the basic principles of the NHS itself: i.e. that the service should be free at the point of use and paid out of general taxation. I think the challenge to local managers and professionals is clear, and success, in my view, imperative.

Chairman: Thank you very much, Dr Mitchell, for another first-class contribution.

6

Commissioning care

PROFESSOR LOU OPIT

I could have summarized my paper with four lines from T.S. Eliot, which seem appropriate to the whole meeting. They are: 'Between the idea and the reality; between the motion and the act falls the shadow.'

This meeting is ostensibly to review progress in the implementation of the White Paper, *Working for Patients*. My task is to deal with the commissioning of services. Since, in my view, neither the White Paper nor any of the subsequent working papers or other documents provide any clear operational guidelines about what commissioning actually is supposed to mean, or more importantly, how it is to be done, I think it is necessary to locate the notion of commissioning within the general ideological context of the policy which the White Paper contains.

The need for commissioning—or for some sort of commissioning anyway—arises out of the intention to create an internal market in the NHS while preserving most of its basic structure. I think probably what Rudolf Klein would have called 'gutting the building and keeping the facade'! The method of generating this market really had three elements in it. These are all well known to you, I am sure, but it is important to remind you of them. The first was to separate administratively and managerially, within every District Health Authority (DHA), their responsibility for obtaining health care on behalf of residents, from their responsibility of providing the actual service components of that care. Secondly, to encourage and to allow for the development of existing hospitals or provider units as organizations for which no DHA was responsible. And thirdly, to encourage or to facilitate the capacity of general practitioners to make direct arrangements for the supply of and payment for certain clinical services as direct contracts between themselves and provider units. Thus was the internal market to be born.

A direct consequence of this separation of responsibility, therefore, was the need for every DHA to be able to specify the Health Service needs for all or most of its resident population in advance and to formulate these needs as contracts with nominated providers. In many ways this step of specifying the health care needs of a population in service-provider terms is fundamental to the whole operation of this artificially created and defined market, and almost every other step has some dependence on it. Thus the contract with providers, the providers' business plans, the rhetoric about quality, are all predicated upon achieving a commissioning process that makes sense. The strange division between core and non-core services is itself a reflection of the limitations in this process of commissioning.

With due respect to Sir Donald Acheson, it is quite clear to me that the Department of Health in official or unofficial guidance to date appears to have no clear idea about what commissioning means, except in ideological terms. In an effort to review the progress—which I thought to be my job—I went to as many official publications as I could stand to read! An example is in the recent document called *Contracts for Health Service* issued by the NHS Management Executive in September 1989 and mysteriously given the sub-title 'Operational principles'. It throws, for me, no light whatsoever on the technology of commissioning services; except, I may say, to state the obvious. Namely, that 'patterns of service provision will be largely influenced by the current pattern of patient referrals'. This whole document has the flavour of a Kafka novel as the content of consecutive paragraphs twists deviously to face both directions at the same time! There is a wonderful section—I think section 3·8—which is about how you deal with the fact that GPs are given the right of where to refer their patients but the districts have no obligation to provide this right for them.

It is at least likely, to me, that the authors of this document had little idea about what the process of commissioning entails, or of the consequences of many of the suggestions they make. In October 1989 the Public Finance Foundation published a document which was entitled *Commissioning Health Services: contract funding in the NHS*. Now I classify this as unofficial Department of Health material and I regard it, again, as an entirely non-prescriptive set of definitions, conditions, and constraints really provided for tiny tots. This is what the new words mean and this is what you are supposed to do. But again, anybody taking this document and attempting to move forward to make a district provide a commissioning mechanism, would get absolutely no help. I find the style of these documents increasingly to be very, very strange. I only wish there was time for some textual analysis. I cannot decide whether they are being unbelievably naïve or fiendishly clever! I am very inclined to the former, but since I have been watching *Yes Minister* and *Yes Prime Minister* this rather drives me to believe the latter!

Another document which I found extraordinarily interesting was a recently issued document from the information technology division of the Department of Health which was called *A framework for information and information technology: a working paper*. This document certainly reveals the scope of the problem: the authors are quite honest about the difficulties as far as data collecting and data use within the NHS is concerned. But as with all the other documents that have come out about information technology in particular, it ends up with an Utopian look forward, except that we are not going to have 30 years to achieve the brave new world. We are now going to take four years to do it. Two other interesting things about that document: the first is the implicit cost of the programme—on the back of an envelope I estimated what this programme was going to cost. I decided that in future outpatients' costs of information were probably greater than the unit cost of the consultant physician. The second thing is that the actual structure of the strategy is based on invoicing. That's what it's for: it's for sending bills. So we are going to be spending £250m-odd to send bills. This seems hardly to be consistent with much of the rhetoric of the White Paper.

So overall, one has to say that out of the increasing output of official and unofficial word factories you see little progress in defining or specifying the logic or the logistics of the commissioning process. Often these documents merely reiterate the irreconcilable nature of much of the White Paper rhetoric. Now at the same time we have, all over the country, consortia, working parties, and consultative groups that are pondering commissioning. How many millions of pounds and thousands of hours of management time have been spent? To what avail? I know not.

In my region, as is traditional, management consultants—being the ultimate repository of wisdom—have been employed to solve the problem! If their provisional report is anything to go by, they have failed to produce anything but a mouse! I also recently wrote to eight regional directors of public health to discover what directions the commissioning process was taking at the regional coal face. I think I somewhat unwisely assumed that regional directors of public health would know. Four failed to reply, three replied but indicated in various ways that very little progress had been made, and the fourth, acknowledging how difficult it was, did claim to have made some progress and to be at the forefront of developments. Unfortunately I did not have time to go and interview those persons concerned but I hope to do so. Thus, from what I have been able to discover, the commissioning of services remains to all intents and purposes a mysterious process. The obvious fact that the *prospective* commissioning of health services is a complex, political, sociological, professional, intellectual, and technical exercise has mainly failed to emerge so far from the information available to me. I have it on good authority now—I cannot reveal the source—that the purpose of the White Paper is being redefined as merely creating a serious debate about health care, rather than a blueprint for Utopia! Now in this case we would have to give it credit for success, for it certainly has promoted a lot of debate!

In line with this new purpose of the White Paper, I want to do something more constructive towards thinking about a feasible commissioning process and where this might lead. I think we can entirely discount the rhetoric of need as it applies to commissioning. The health care need of a given population, a phrase which figures extensively in documents, is a complex, even a contentious notion for many elements of need. Because the concepts of health care needs are so ill-defined and because we have so little information related to needs other than that which expresses itself as a demand for services, and that is already modified and defined by clinicians, I think we have to abandon the notion of need for the purposes of commissioning altogether. In short, we do not know and we will probably never know what the need is for care for varicose veins, pneumonia, menorrhagia, or thousands of other problems. We know something about the incidence of some diseases, such as malignancy or congenital defects. But even here the information we most often require is prevalence and not incidence, since people are often treated more than once. Even this does not forecast demand in service terms. Knowing about how much illness exists and using this to infer the service needs is an extraordinarily difficult step. Neither does the sort of data about incidence or prevalence encapsulate properly the very complex, negotiable relationship between the disease itself and the indications for its care. Every clinician of any experience knows this. Little difficulties, such as effectiveness or outcome, also intrude into the concept of need.

Available information bases are restricted mainly to expressed demand, and for many of these clinically specified demands we know in detail only about the demand that has been met. In other words, we know something about the illness type or treatment of those who are discharged from hospital, but information about those on the waiting list or those who attend the out-patients or emergency department is far more restricted. About those whose need has not been expressed we know virtually nothing. So we quickly reach the point of recognizing that our commissioning mechanism has to be based on measures of expressed demand for all its inadequacies. In theory some such data are available everywhere through the existing regional and district information systems. The problem is how to use this complex database to examine and describe the future likely demand for acute services. I think all of you at this stage would ask the same two questions: (1) do we have reliable, relevant, and timely data about expressed demand?;

(2) do we have a typology or a classification which enables us to express this demand in useful ways? Now by 'useful' I mean management-focused, intelligible, and appropriate to commissioning. The ICD9 or 10 were not developed for this purpose and, in my view, they are a positive impediment to management action. It is a great classification for obsessional doctors! In our region I'm afraid we would have to also answer the first question with a resounding 'No'. Our data are of a pretty frightful quality. As for the second question, the answer must be that DRGs are not the answer. I do not have time to outline why DRGs are absolutely useless for the purpose of commissioning, so I must deny myself that pleasure.

What approaches are possible? As I am trying to indicate, to commission health care provision, even when you have accurate, timely, consistent, and reliable data, is a really tricky business. On the one hand, if we only commission large blocks of clinical work as block contracts across or within specialties, the theory of competitive commissioning—which the White Paper promotes—will become nearly meaningless. While on the other hand, detailed commissioning for specific illnesses or procedure groups requires good information and will appear to imply a clinical knowledge and a technical competence which commissioning authorities will not have. In addition, we have another little problem. Commissioning procedures directly—which is very much part of the flavour of the commissioning notion—is also likely to increase intervention rates and to favour operative over non-operative solutions to clinical problems. This is precisely the problem which fee-for-service medical payment systems have and which in turn led to the DRGs as cost-containment technology.

It is not the commissioning *per se* which is problematic but the need to convert a commission into a contract. The difficulty and the precision which a contract entails must vary with different levels of commissioning expressed as illness or procedures. This is sufficiently complex to need much thought, discussion, and experiment—before embarking on an inadequately conceived and formulated national programme. It is not merely a problem of data acquisition that we are dealing with or of data interpretation; it is a problem inherent in medical care itself.

I want to try to indicate an alternative approach which I have tried to develop. I don't know that my region is very interested in it; I'm not sure how many people understand it. I think I'm found to be quite difficult to deal with anyway, but I did try to look at this problem in a realistic way, given the limitations that existed in the world of health care.

If commissioning is intended to be a competitive process, focused on good value and quality, it is necessary to start with the problems which arise in the historically determined present. What worries me about many presentations is that they are completely ahistorical: it is as though the world started last year. It is a bit like adolescents feel about sex: they think sex was invented in 1986! Again, the White Paper managed to avoid this problem completely—there is absolutely no historical context. Our starting point, in the approach that we have tried to think about and develop, is to define and to redefine coherent groups of service types as potential contractor units with whom contracts could be formulated. Now this is actually quite a complicated job since there are often several service alternatives for the care of some illnesses. These represent local outcomes of historical modes of practice and different stages of service development in different districts or different hospitals. You can find lots of examples: in some places if you look at the work load of the thoracic medicine unit or the general medical unit you will find they are substantially sharing large elements of the case-load. In some districts you will find plastic surgery, general surgery, orthopaedics, or urology contributing variously to the provision of care of a number of different problems. It raises very critical issues at the outset of the commissioning and contracting process. Questions like: 'Should general surgeons carry out urological procedures? Who should perform the excision and repair of large skin tumours? Who should repair severed flexor tendons?' Now these are very tricky questions and the answers are fraught with problems which we doubt are within the competence and skill of a health authority to decide. They do, however, require answers if commissioning is to have the meaning or the effect intended by the White Paper. So we try to address this question, at least as an agenda item, in political discussion in terms of individual districts.

The next step is to define a set of operational acute service goals and, associated with this, a set of pathways to care. It is not possible for me to do other than to provide a brief sketch. The principle of our approach then—and we think a principle of all approaches—needs to be as follows. Demand data from any single District Health Authority is difficult to interpret sensibly since we have no clear logic to formulate expected need. Local demand may reflect a bewildering variety of local factors including boundary flows, demographic and socioeconomic conditions, previous levels of provision and methods of practice. You can confirm this very easily by looking at the wide range of treatment rates, say in surgical specialties, between different districts. In almost every case we do not know what the correct rate of treatment is for some procedure, even if that concept is meaningful. In some situations and for some procedures there are clearly age-related effects, but in many others this is not an explanation of the variation. The other feasible approach then is to examine the relationship between various factors and outputs for all districts having a given service or service mix. In other words, you cannot simply look at a single district—a single district's data can be meaningless.

In carrying out such analysis, we assume the existence of an overriding normative demand based on demographic and socioeconomic factors. This enables us at least to recognize outliers as exceptional. In this way then we can derive an expected normal demand level within any particular service goal. The critical interaction between demand and supply is, in large measure, still not addressed. We have actually applied this now for our region in urology, general surgery, trauma and orthopaedic surgery, and for plastic surgery. It is a possible basis for commissioning in these specialties. Now when we have reached this point, we come to the question of how detailed the commissioning process should be and this emerges, again, as a serious problem. Which case-mix elements should be specified in detail? Which in large blocks? What should be regarded as core? What do we do about secondary or tertiary referrals between specialists or specialties? It is at this point that we require the development of methods of specifying case-mix, both for reasons of commissioning and to derive measures of case-mix complexity. Initially, like many others, we pinned our hopes on DRGs as the appropriate model, but problems with the typology, the software and the basic structure of the classification led us to explore alternatives.

Now I do not have time to do much more, only to specify what I think of as three principles of the commissioning analysis. These are:

1. That commissioning should specify the expected distribution of illness within some broadly defined and usable typology—that is, neither ICD nor DRGs.

2. Procedures commissioned should always be formulated within the illness or problem type—not as separate elements

3. Medical audit should be seen as part and parcel of the commissioning process: this seems critical to me. In many respects, what comes out of the commissioning analyses are questions which will feed back into the medical audit system, and from which we can obtain technical arguments or excuses.

Finally, I think we can be certain that whatever form the commissioning and contracting process takes, there is a need for complete, reliable, consistent, and timely data about demand and the methods available to make this information usable for management—and that is one of our key problems. We seem a great distance away from this objective, and in the end we may lose it altogether. There is a risk, I believe, that unrealistic, complex, irrelevant, opportunistic, and extravagant technologies—mostly from the USA—focused on audit or on resource management, will be widely and badly implemented. This, when the existing data capture and analytical systems are still inadequate to provide any usable base for commissioning.

Titmuss, in a paper titled *Community Care—Fact or Fiction?* stated in 1963 that if '...English social history is any guide, confusion has often been the mother of complacency. In the public mind the aspirations of reformers are transmitted by the touch of a phrase, into hard-won reality. What some hope will one day exist is suddenly thought by many to exist already'. I believe that we have witnessed this to an extreme degree with White Paper documents and thinking.

Finally, I would like to finish with an Indian fable. This is a fable which concerns a centipede. This poor centipede had arthritis in every one of its hundred legs. It was extraordinarily miserable. One day the centipede was put in touch with a very, very wise old owl—who I may say had been a health economist before he became a wise old owl! He went to the wise old owl and he said: 'Mr Owl, I have this awful, unbelievable suffering. Please, is there something you can do for me.' The wise old owl reflected, and he said, 'Yes, I believe there is something I can do. What you need to do is to turn into a human being, then you will only have two legs and the suffering will be correspondingly reduced by a factor of 50.' The centipede was absolutely delighted by this and he hobbled away with plans to put this programme in place. When he got home he realized he had forgotten to ask the owl something important. So next day he went back to see the wise old owl. He said, 'Yesterday I was so excited with the wonderful news that you brought me that I forgot to ask you how to do it. How do I turn into a man?' At this the owl became very uppity. He said, 'Look here, Mr Centipede! My job is the policy; your job is the implementation.'

Chairman: Thank you very much, Lou. You are not only entertaining and critical, but also extremely constructive and helpful. Thank you very much.

7

Discussion

Dr Michael Joffe: I was very interested to hear the contributions on audit and needs assessment. The question I want to ask is: what future does either have in policy making under the internal market?

A few months ago the Social Services Committee published its comments on the White Paper. It was widely reported that these were critical of the White Paper, primarily because of the lack of adequate data on costs. In other words, the more that one gets into the detail of how things work, the more one gets concerned with costs to the exclusion of everything else. Particularly when the rest of the data, for example, on audit and assessment of needs, is less accessible to managers. I fear that costs will come to dominate everything and that this will mirror in the Health Service what we have seen in British Industry, which is dominated by costs containment rather than research, development, and training. It is my anxiety that we will see an overall decline in standards.

Chairman: If I could just say before we answer the question that cost has been dominating health care as long as I have been in the Department and will not suddenly begin to dominate it in 1991.

Professor Raymond Hoffenberg: I think things would be very much worse without some audit.

Professor Lou Opit: There is an irreconcilable rhetoric in the White Paper because it starts with the idea of a fixed, finite amount of money. It also talks about needs, but it is not going to provide any additional money to meet the needs, so it is basically about a system of rationing. The whole debate since 1974 in the Department of Health and in Government, has been characterized by the fact that we gave up the idea of meeting needs. The Regional Allocation Working Party

(RAWP) was the beginning of it. We went to the idea of rationing. That remains and in fact will be stiffened.

Chairman: Yes, and I think most countries that do not have rationing are trying to get it. Would you agree?

Professor Lou Opit: Well possibly, yes.

Chairman: Thank you—I've scored one point!

Dr Ian Greatorex: I, like Deirdre Cunningham, work in an inner city area with lots of problems. I was interested in her attempts to assess needs and in how she, in a Department of Public Health Medicine, is trying to speak to the people who live in her district about their demands. I am thinking of community development approaches which, it seems to me, we also need in addition to traditional epidemiology.

Dr Deirdre Cunningham: Yes, we certainly are planning to talk to the public. Let me give you the example of our heart disease needs-assessment project. We do not feel that demand is synonymous with needs because the public do not demand the preventive and screening services which we feel we ought to be providing. What we have done is to divide the natural history of the disease into seven stages which we have agreed with those who provide prevention and treatment services. We have set up a Parkside Heart Disease Prevention Group involving clinicians, the health promotion unit, dieticians, general practitioners, and managers. One of our first projects is a survey of general practitioners and of the public to find out what their requirements are. We are feeling our way on this, and in the first contracting period we will not have gone very far down the road.

Dr Donald Richardson: Could I begin by thanking everyone concerned for the quality of the papers presented. I think they have been absolutely magnificent and have provided a great deal for all of us to think about, both in our daily clinical practice as well as for those of us who have responsibility on health authorities for implementing the White Paper.

Every contribution, I think, has raised endless questions. I would like to highlight one or two. Dr Parston and Professor Opit paint a picture which I recognize from implementing the White Paper in general practice. I am thankful that I am not intending to go in for direct contracting myself when I think of the difficulties which are going to be compounded in general practice.

That we have been destabilized is unquestionable. Many of us, as the President of the Royal College of General Practitioners has said, have been demotivated. Two contributions today—Professor Hoffenberg and Dr Cunningham—talked about the necessity of knowing what you are doing. I am bound to say that I am not at all sure that I know what I am going to be doing after 1 April 1990. In addition to doing what I have done over many years, there is an added requirement to see all new patients, all patients I haven't seen for three years, and the over-75 year olds every year. There is no indication of what resources will be available to deal with what I may find nor, indeed, the anticipated outcome of all this activity. I am not sure about the value of measuring the height of adults and taking blood pressures in children. I think that this is an unfortunate diversion of my time and that of my staff from many other, more worthwhile objectives. To me this is a matter of substantial regret.

Dr Ruth Owen: Dr Mitchell, in your contrasting of the successful and unsuccessful Canadian organizations, it struck me that many of the features in the unsuccessful organizations had a lot in common with the White Paper one year on—particularly the lack of knowledge, the lack of information and the confusion. Did you intend this?

Dr John Mitchell: I don't think that the White Paper has yet significantly affected the way hospitals manage their health care outcome, although it has caused a lot of concern and speculation. The point I was trying to make was that the agenda for the White Paper implementation is not necessarily the same as the agenda for the people who deliver health care. We should start safeguarding the health of our communities by having a clear idea of what our health care organizations are about and what they should deliver.

Dr M. Impallomeni: I would like to disagree with Professor Opit who says that contracting out is something which is not yet happening. The first impact of the White Paper has already occurred. Contracting out is already happening in geriatric medicine where the privatization of long-stay wards is occurring all over the country. This results from the fact that under the White Paper any resident of a nursing home on 1 April 1991 will attract income support benefit. If, therefore, the District Health Authority sells the site of the long-stay hospital to a private company in order to have a private nursing home built, the patients would be classed as residents in a private nursing home from that date. They will then attract income support to the tune of £200 per week. In the case of our Health Authority this involves 72 long-stay patients, which amounts to £800 000 per annum—half the current over-expenditure. So I wonder what the panel thinks we should do, as clinicians, to introduce some element of planning, taking into consideration the needs of our elderly population.

Dr Greg Parston: There are no answers, obviously, but I do think that one can look at what health authorities are trying to do, to ensure that hospital services do not dominate the provision of care. We see community units, for example, beginning to talk about themselves becoming the commissioning agencies. We see health authorities beginning to talk in terms of evolving into health maintenance organizations. Clinicians are becoming very much involved and defining, I say with respect, a very different kind of commissioning agency from that which Professor Opit described. The latter I take to mean a health service insurance company. The former are health assurance companies and, in so far as clinicians want to guarantee a continuity of care beyond the hospital, that health assurance area is where you must become committed and involved.

Dr Gleeson: I would like to ask Professor Hoffenberg how he envisages the development of extra time to devote to medical audit. We in Jersey are trying to get audit meetings going and we are finding it very difficult even to get junior doctors to the meetings on time because of the pressure of the clinical work. It is certainly a worthwhile exercise, but the practicalities of getting it introduced seem to me quite considerable.

Professor Hoffenberg: Thank you very much. I do agree with you. In Birmingham we held our meetings at a regular weekly lunch hour and the hospital very generously provided sandwiches and coffee. I think that is very helpful because people do usually break for lunch. You are asking a lot from doctors to give up their traditional time and I am sure that Sir Donald would agree that something has to be done to find that extra time. This will, as I said, need more appointments.

Mr Croft: It seems to me that the split into purchaser and provider functions will multiply the need for good-calibre managers by a factor of three or four. First of all, does the panel agree? Secondly, where will they all come from? Thirdly, where will the cash to pay for them come from?

Dr John Mitchell: Yes, I think you are right, but that is not new. I think we have been aware of the lack of management capability around the Health Service for a good many years and the White Paper just brings that to the fore.

I have no direct answer to the question, except to make the observation that professionals presently spend a lot of time managing their health services without recognizing that this is what they are doing. One of the ways of improving and enlarging the management capability is to involve doctors and other professionals more effectively in management.

Dr Greg Parston: I can suggest answers to your three questions. Yes. The United States. And, your pocket.

Dr Peter Fletcher: An excellent series of papers this morning I thought, but as a negative, fearful clinician I wonder if I could ask Professor Opit to make explicit what I thought was implicit in his fable. That is, if the owl's policy is implemented, surely you are going to convert a centipede into a human—which is excellent, of course—but you are going to end up with a two-legged creature that cannot walk rather than a hundred-legged creature that cannot walk—not a very good outcome in audit terms!

Professor Lou Opit: The answer is 'Yes'.

Chairman: The answers are getting shorter! There is only one shorter one, and that is 'No'.

Dr Peter Jaffe: May I just swap quotes with Professor Opit. I thought he was going to quote: 'Things fall apart, that the centre cannot hold'!

The major central role is clearly going to lie with the purchasing agencies, which will have a very contentious role in deciding priorities; the most value-laden, the most political, and the least discussed. Furthermore, managers seem to be the least interested in that particular area. How can one develop sufficient interest and discussion of the purchaser's role and how can the clinician get involved in the value judgements that are going to be implicit in that?

Chairman: Could I just say that there has recently been a one-day conference on the role of the District Health Authority, and other such meetings are planned. This is a very important function and that fact will need to be emphasized.

Professor Lou Opit: Yes, I completely agree. The whole system, in theory at least, is driven by the commissioning purchasing system. That sets the priorities; that in essence will determine what the providers actually do.

Your second point: I am seriously alarmed about the absence of clinicians in any of the debates about commissioning and the development of models. I believe it is essential that a coherent, clinical voice is heard at regional, at district, as well as national levels.

Dr Bobbie Jacobson: On the purchasing side, we have worked out that locally we will probably need at least 7000 different contracts to cover a condition-led approach. I was therefore very interested in what Lou Opit had to say. Given that we are being pressed to think ahead to 1992, we should perhaps focus on one or two fundamental questions. Is the internal market necessary to push forward some of the very key issues that have been raised in terms of assessing the health needs of the local population? If not, what should we be advising future governments to do about health and health care beyond 1992?

Dr Greg Parston: I do not think the internal market is necessary. Some spirit of enterprise and perhaps competition can be fostered in ways other than through the internal market. What is necessary is to be explicit about what we are doing and I think that is one of the great advantages of the White Paper. There is an attempt to link performance to outcome and, however difficult that is, for the first time we are beginning to get people thinking about what they are doing.

What do you advise the Government to do? What *I* would do is not be concerned about what you tell them you are doing, but what you begin getting people within your locality to think about doing. I have argued for a long time that the confusion at the centre is fantastic because it lets you, at the local level, run with it. You should just take it and run with it.

Dr Margaret Judd: It has been fascinating listening to this morning's papers but I am a little concerned that we have only been looking at the English-speaking nations. I am not a particularly committed European, but I gather that most of our partners in the Common Market are in a similar position as regards cost containment. I wonder if Sir Donald would like to make any comment on the future in that respect.

Chairman: All I would wish to say is that I believe that there is no country in the world that is not anxious about its expenditure, whether it is the United States or whatever other country it might be. In Europe I think the striking things are the great variety of systems of health care: all of them are under scrutiny and criticism, and most of them are more expensive than ours.

Dr Keith Baker: This question is particularly directed to Dr Cunningham. We have talked about needs assessment. We, as health authorities, have a responsibility to improve the health of the population. If our needs assessment leads us to believe that the most useful application of our resources is outside the provision of health services, and to employ those resources in other ways, what freedom do you think the new purchaser/provider separation will allow us to do so?

Dr Deirdre Cunningham: This will remain a problem at least until we stop managing hospitals units directly. How future districts will interpret their roles in purchasing health care outside this system I am not quite sure. I would have thought alternatives such as housing are valid options.

Chairman: Looking a decade or two ahead, if the District Health Authority is to improve the health of the population for which it is responsible, the question which will be asked is whether health care is the best place to put the money or whether somewhere else is more appropriate?

Sir Terence English: If, as Dr Parston has suggested, there is confusion at the centre and events are left to develop at the periphery, my question to Dr Cunningham is: come this time next year, how much conformity does she expect to see in the definition of local health needs by the 192 health districts up and down the country?

Dr Deirdre Cunningham: At the moment I see considerable disarray. I do not think there will be very much conformity at all. When I mentioned that my nightmare is that every district will be assessing needs for hip replacements I imagined there would be some common denominator but that the models developed will vary quite widely. In the first year, I imagine most districts will reach the position which Lou Opit has put forward; namely, they will base their first year's purchasing on existing demand. I hope that our network and dissemination of good practice will help us to look at the best ways of estimating need and applying these to our districts. I hope that we will be able to develop basic methods which will allow us to assess needs for particular services. Once developed and disseminated, it will be up to districts to apply those to their own area. We could then say, 'Here is the average way of calculating needs for these particular services; do you require more or less of them?' I think the major problem which we are going to face is when, for instance, we are comparing needs for services for cardiovascular disease with needs for paediatric services, services for elderly people, or other groups. I am sure there are going to be diverse ways of determining where the money and other resources go.

Professor Lou Opit: I just wanted to say that I think it will not only be next year that commissioning will be based on demand. Although we have all these models of the epidemiology of disease from which we are going to forecast the amount of care, I am afraid that this wonderful reductionist fairyland, even if it could be applied to 20 diseases a year, means that for the next 15 years we are still going to say, 'Varicose veins—now how many do we usually do?'

Dr Greg Parston: I would like to just come back, if I may, to the previous question. I think that there is going to be a great deal of freedom for commissioning agencies to spend money on housing, but those commissioning agencies are not going to be District Health Authorities. They are going to be local authorities. It is very silly for us to sit here and think that this White Paper sits in isolation from other White Papers and from other issues that are going on in the public sector generally. Remember that local authorities under *Caring for people* are going to have responsibility for designating where money goes and to whom. They are going to hold a lot of the money that is now spent on community care or the homeless, and that money is not ring-fenced. They can spend the money wherever they like: on the homeless, on roads, on education; wherever they like. If that is the case, then what we end up with is a national hospital service and commissioning agencies buying other services. I think we have to move ahead on this White Paper fully cognisant that there are developments in other White Papers that could significantly and radically change the way in which we regard commissioning agencies and the way in which we regard the provision of care.

Mr Derek McLintock: As we are talking about commissioning at the moment, may I address this particularly to Professor Opit. As a gynaecologist I can see that we have got a lot of abilities, although at present rather inaccurate, in assessing the prevalence and incidence of the diseases that we deal with. I know that Professor Opit has read much more of the White Paper than I have. Have I missed somewhere the possibility that the Government is going to give obstetric clinical directors at least nine months' notification of any increases or decreases in interest rates or even power cuts in a privatized electrical industry?

Chairman: Shall we leave it at that? In which case, may I thank you all for your contributions and thank the speakers again for a very good morning.

Session 2: A seamless service?

PROFESSOR WALTER HOLLAND—Chairman

I welcome you to the after-lunch session. The title I suspect was chosen before this morning's speakers, but at least it does have a question mark.

8

Funding the future

PROFESSOR TONY CULYER

Let me begin with some rather naïve views about the relationship between health care spending, health and the quality of care. One goes like this:

$$Q = M$$

This I call the monetary theory of health quality and I put it in a functional form. It says 'more quality is directly related to the amount of money put in'. Like most mathematical formulations it has a graphical interpretation (Fig. 4). For those of you who find this a bit sophisticated it says, 'the more you put in, the better the quality'. Zero in, zero quality. The relationship is linear and the curve goes on for ever and ever, amen.

An alternative monetary theory of *health* is slightly more sophisticated, at least as far as the vertical axis is concerned. This theory goes like this:

$$H = M$$

This says that 'health is directly related to the amount of money put in'. So again, a functional relationship: the more money you put in, the more health you get out. That, likewise, has a graphical representation (Fig. 5). This at least has a refreshing focus on outcome, which we were reminded we should focus on this morning. Of the three approaches to monitoring quality in health care: structure, process, and outcome—three virtues, rather like Faith, Hope, and Charity—the greatest of them is also undoubtedly the third, outcome.

For either of these two functional representations, more is always better, for ever and ever, amen. There are a lot of reasons why they are not very helpful, although they do represent, implicitly at least, the thinking of many people

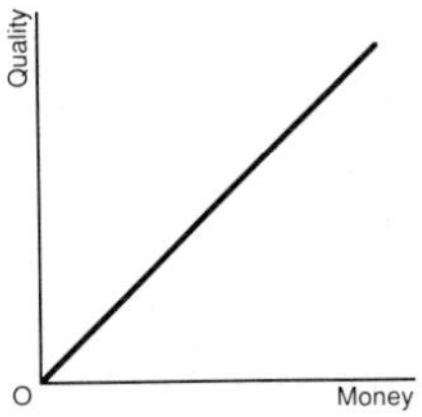

Fig. 4. Monetary relationship between quality of care and health care spending.

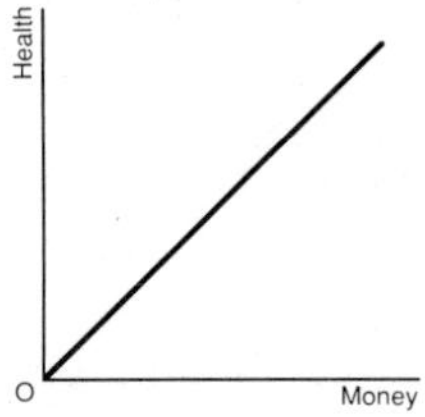

Fig. 5. Alternative monetary relationship between health outcome and health care spending.

about health care. They are not particularly helpful in addressing the sort of question that I want to address, which is: how does one set about thinking, let alone deciding and possibly persuading governments, about what is the appropriate total amount of money to be spent on the National Health Service?

Let us take a step back and ask ourselves about some objectives for health services (Table 4). We get marginally more sophisticated now. I suggest that there are five major goals that most health systems seek to satisfy. These are:

1. a socially fair distribution of services, or of health itself. This is subject to some interpretation as to what fairness, equity, or justice might mean in the context of health—but generally speaking this is one objective.

2. effective and efficient medical practice.

3. clinical freedom from government interference.

4. freedom from interference in pricing and pay.

5. budgetary and expenditure control.

Now unfortunately, God has ordained that you cannot have all of these five desiderata at the same time—you must choose.

DESIDERATA					
Socially fair distribution	**Effective and efficient medical practice**	**Clinical freedom from government interference**	**Freedom from interference in pricing and pay**	**Budgetary and expenditure control**	**Prototypical system**
YES	YES	YES	YES	YES	Nirvana
YES	YES	YES	YES	NO	The provider's dream
YES	YES	NO	NO	YES	The NHI/NHS dream
NO	?	YES	YES	NO	Laissez-faire competitive system
NO	?	Y/N	Y/N	NO	USA

Table 4. Objectives for health services

I have suggested some alternative ways in which different people might dream about things. The provider's dream is: 'Yes, of course we want all these criteria, but we do not want anybody to control expenditure' so we can go on spending, for ever and ever, amen.

The first dream is of course that of Nirvana, which is out—alas! That is the one that the Americans seek, as it is every American's native-born right to seek Nirvana. But of course they fail and what they have is actually a mess. They certainly do not have a socially fair distribution; there are some 30 million uninsured Americans not eligible for Medicare or Medicaid and a further 20-odd million who are severely and seriously under-insured.

There is a question mark about whether or not medical practice in the US is effective and efficient—it depends what they are being effective and efficient *at*. If it is a question of meeting *needs* then the US system has some of the very best and some of the very worst examples. If it is a question of meeting *demands* then it may do a little better, provided you do not worry about those in need who are unable to express a demand.

Clinical freedom? Well, to some extent. In the US Medicare programme, as a consequence of DRGs, there is substantial lack of freedom in many respects both for managers and for clinicians. In other sectors, considerable more freedom exists. Again it is a mixture. Likewise with freedom from interference in pricing and pay—it depends which bit of the American system you are in. Budgetary and expenditure control? By Jove, they've tried! They have invested in many techniques of control over the years but one of the remarkable things is that if you look at the curve of expenditure over time, it goes on, ever upwards, for ever and ever, amen.

What *we* aspire to is, I presume, what I have called the National Health Insurance or the National Health Service dream. In pursuing this we seem prepared partially to compromise two kinds of freedom. I am assuming we really do aspire to the first two desiderata, but our performance really puts a question mark over our success in attaining the third and fourth. Like the Americans, we aspire to something but we do not really quite achieve it. Our system is, however, certainly socially fairer than theirs and we have also effectively controlled overall spending where they have failed dismally.

Now, where you stand on these desiderata always depends on where you sit. If you are a provider, you might take one view; if you are a clinician you might take another; if you are a manager, a politician, or whatever, yet other views.

The way we are going to try to achieve these goals in the post-White Paper world, is essentially threefold. Through cash-limited budgets to ensure budgetary and expenditure control. We are also going to have population-based budget allocations plus zero or small user charges, to maintain some sort of fairness in access terms (at least on the pricing side). Finally, the big thing that we are all concerned about today: market competition between providers to achieve effectiveness and efficiency. The conditions for a market to be efficient are horrendously difficult to sustain and require enormous political courage. One of the reasons why I suspect that the White Paper is not going to accomplish the dream of its inventors is because they will not ultimately have the political courage to push through what is necessary in order to achieve it. It certainly implies a greater degree of managerial control over clinical practice, through medical audit and a variety of other measures discussed today, as well as greater local discretion over pricing and pay. This may of course have the net effect of increasing expenditure without any corresponding increase in output. But it also requires much local discretion in pricing and investment strategies, genuine openness in the bidding process, sufficient information to be able to monitor contract performance and, ultimately, the possibility of exit for the unsuccessful providers, even if they are within the public sector.

The issue that I really want to talk about is how do we judge the adequacy, both now and in the future, of the level of expenditure of the Health Service. The trouble with those two quantity theories that I looked at earlier is familiar to you. Quality is identified with the *quantity* of staffing, equipment, capital and so on, and the *inherent* input quality—like embodiment of the latest technologies and qualifications of staff. It is not related to the quality of *outcome*. You will probably be familiar with the work of the Office of Technology Assessment of the United States which estimates that only around 20 per cent of commonly used procedures in medical care are of proven effectiveness and an even smaller percentage of those are of proven cost-effectiveness. Similar estimates have been made by other individuals, like Kerr-White and Archie Cochrane.

Secondly, of course, the link between health and health care is complex, lagged, and influenced by many other factors. As Lou Opit reminded us this morning, history is important. History is important in assessing outcome because it determines where you start off from in terms of health, as well as what the possibilities are for doing anything about it. However, whatever the link between health and health care, it is certainly not simply linear. This is a simple but important point to bear in mind. I interpret the fundamental theory which lies behind the White Paper to be essentially a modified sort of this simple input/output approach that I illustrated at the beginning. The thinking behind the White Paper suggests that the current relationship looks more like that in figure 6. We might interpret the health axis more sophisticatedly, so as to reflect the problems that many people alluded to this morning. Please note that the appropriate measure of outcome is the *change* in health. It is not your actual level of mortality; it is the difference between what mortality would have been before and after the introduction of the particular intervention. It is not actual morbidity; it is the difference that interventions make to morbidity. It is not actual levels of functioning of individuals; it is the difference between what their functioning would have been and what it has become as a result of, or what it is believed it will become with, an intervention. But there are diminishing returns. Following a phase of productive health care, you have the flat of the curve medicine—to use the words of a well-known US health economist, Victor Fuchs. Beyond that you have medical iatrogenesis, Ivan Illich's medical nemesis.

I conjecture that the Government's thinking is that, wherever we are on the outcome curve, the service comprises a mixture of different procedures. Some of these have a high slope and are marginally very productive; some are pretty flat and do not make much difference; and some may actually be harmful. Very frequently we do not know one from the other. If we could get the system to address these issues more systematically and provide, via better identificarion of needs by

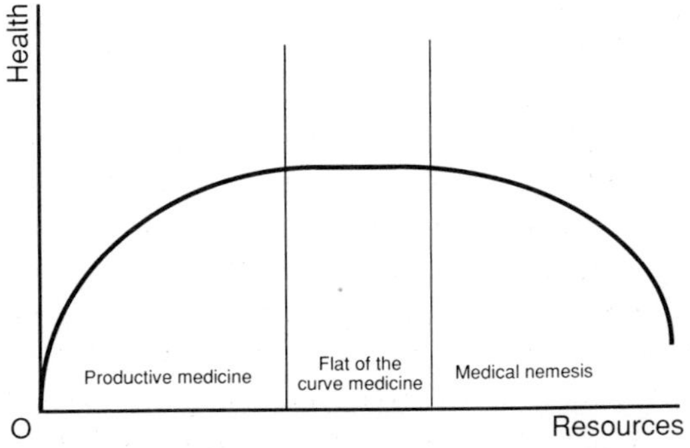

Fig. 6. Relationship between health outcome and resource input.

Authorities and via competition between providers, a general environment conducive to efficiency and productivity, we will then get rid of the inefficient aspects of the service. We would increase the slope of this curve so that we get one that looks like the heavily drawn curve in figure 7. This is what the White Paper is intended to accomplish.

So, here is a kind of post-White Paper idealized production function of health. God only knows if internal markets can produce this wonder. Let us assume that the miracle happens, so that one real political fear of throwing good money after bad has been removed. The only remaining question is: how much should we spend? How many resources should we be putting in here? Where on the heavy curve in figure 7 should we try to locate expenditure?

There are a couple of standard ways in which this sort of question has been addressed in the past, and they are pretty poor. One with which you will be familiar is the international comparisons of spending per head of population. I have compared 15 European countries with their spending per head in US dollars in purchasing power parity (Fig. 8). If we had straight exchange rates the differences would look even more dramatic than they do there. As you can see Britain is twelfth out of the fifteen, spending about 60 per cent of the rate that Sweden spends per head. Obviously, you say looking at that, we are not spending enough. But if you rank these countries in terms of their income per head of population you would find

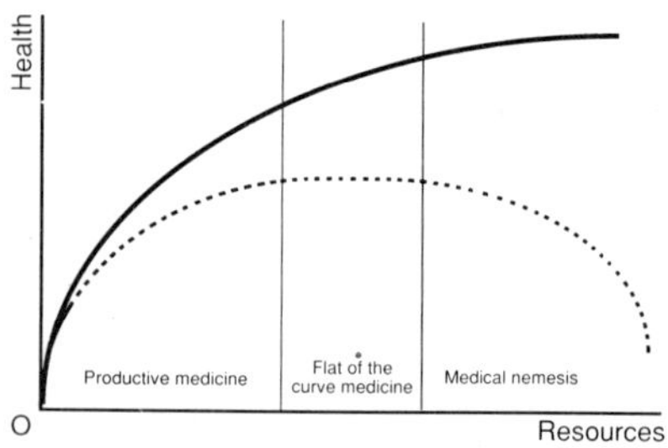

Fig. 7. Postulated future relationship between health outcome and resource input.

that they rank in much the same way. You must not forget that Britain is a relatively poor country. Let us therefore make an adjustment for income. If we do a regression of Gross Domestic Product per head and the per head expenditure on health services for the Organization of Economic Co-operation and Development countries, we get a relationship between spending per head and income per head, shown in figure 9. If you were par for the course, given your income level, you would need to be on the line. The per caput UK income was then about £8500. Lo and behold, we are spending less than the line predicts: therefore the Health Service is underfunded.

Now these are two fairly familiar ways of looking at international comparisons. Both of these approaches are problematic. After all, why assume that what the others are doing is right? Most of these other countries—particularly the high-spending ones—are obsessed about cost-containment and actually believe that they spend too much. What you get for your health care dollar is quite variable from country to country. For example, Germany is 15 per cent richer than the British per head of population using purchasing power parity measures; richer still if you use ordinary exchange rates. It

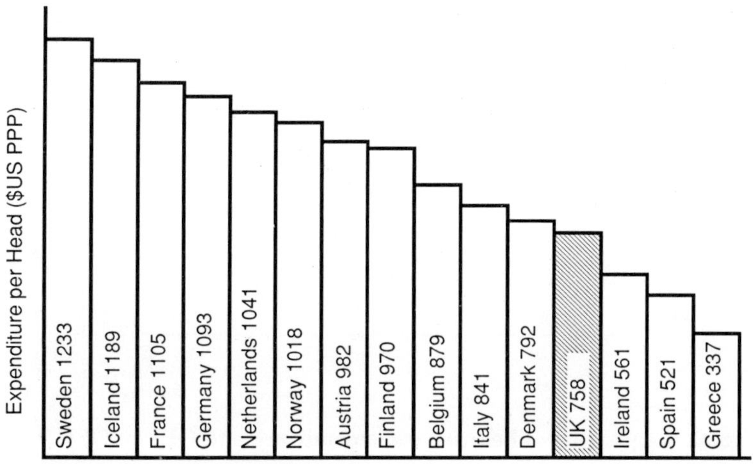

Fig. 8. Health care expenditure per head in 1987 for various countries.

actually spends 44 per cent more per head on health care than we do, but it has 59 per cent fewer nurses than the UK. It has considerably more doctors than we have and it pays them considerably more than we do. The United States is 40 per cent richer per head and spends twice as much per head on health care as we do. It has, however, 27 per cent fewer hospital beds, with very short lengths of stay, and 30 per cent fewer nurses per head of population than the UK. So the mixture of major and costly inputs varies from country to country. You really need to look beyond the financial figures. In the end, we are forced to ask about the productivity and efficiency of the resources used in health care and their value when used in this manner compared to their value in other uses.

I do not know what you understand by efficiency, but there are three quite distinct meanings to the word (Table 5). The first is that you do not use more resources than are necessary to achieve your aim. Any particular aim can usually be achieved by using a variety of resources—for example, as we have just considered, different mixes of doctors and nurses—so

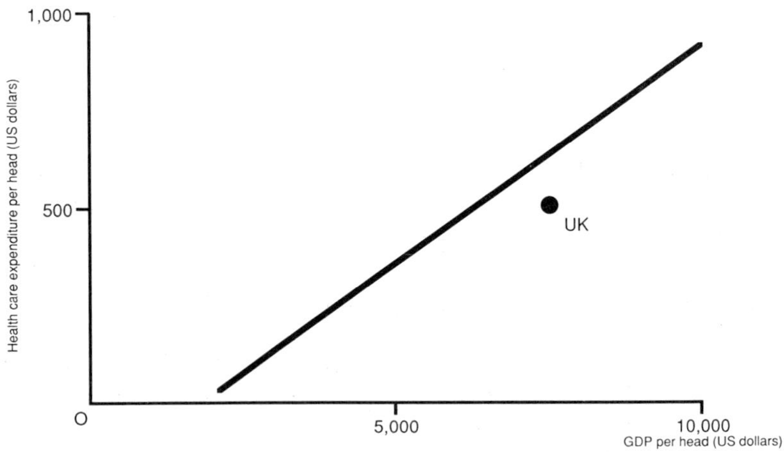

Fig. 9. Regression of health care expenditure and GDP of OECD countries 1981.

there are normally a variety of ways of achieving particular objectives that meet this first criterion. The second one is not incurring a greater cost than is necessary to achieve your aim. You take account of the costs of the alternative bundles that are efficient in the first sense and the least cost one is the cost-effective one. The third notion of efficiency combines the first two and adds: attaining an appropriate rate of throughput or output, which implies attaining an appropriate level of overall expenditure.

Table 5. Different meanings of efficiency

1. Not using more resources than are necessary to achieve your aim.
2. Not incurring a greater cost than is necessary to achieve your aim.
3. Meaning 2 plus attaining an appropriate rate of throughput or output.

It should be clear that if the White Paper is going to do anything in the way of efficiency, it addresses only the first two of these three concepts. It has really nothing to say about the third. It is devoid of any statements about how one assesses the appropriate overall level of spending, which is crucial if we are going to get an efficient sized health-care sector. It seems clear, however, that improving efficiency in the first two senses is a necessary condition for further substantial injections of real resources. The Government clearly needs to be satisfied that extra resources will not be swallowed up in relatively inefficient activity, or in higher pay with no increase in productivity. In order to convince Government, as well as ourselves, a combination is required of 'hard heads and soft hearts'. We need hard heads to confront the issues involved in evaluating effectiveness and cost-effectiveness of clinical procedures, and soft hearts in ensuring that the ultimate test of effectiveness is in terms of patient well-being. This will need a lot of thinking about, clarifying meanings, doing the appropriate trials, and making well-based judgements about cost-effectiveness.

There will be lots of room for disagreement about what is enough, even when we have thought through these issues and done lots of measurements. But I think, provided the sources of disagreement can be identified, one may be at least on the way to presenting cases more effectively than they have been in the past. I suspect that, fundamentally, the differences between people about what is enough overall hinge on disagreements about issues shown in Table 6. What are the objectives? I have tended, in my interpretation of the White Paper, to assume that objectives are health-related. Now, I may be wrong. And even if health promotion were the main business of the health service it is not necessarily its only business. There are other important things that health services do, like providing information, caring, reassuring, and so on. A balance of those things is clearly something which one can discuss. The priorities that you put upon them relative to other uses of public money can vary: is it more important to have some marginal increase in health, supposing we agree what that means, or more defence or education, or private consumption, or... ?

Table 6. Disagreements about what is 'enough' (for efficiency and equity) probably derive from more fundamental disagreements about:

1. objectives;
2. what it is to be efficient;
3. what it is to be equitable;
4. the best institutional framework for accomplishing the above.

I have given three definitions of efficiency which are at least mutually consistent, but there are a lot of loose notions of efficiency around about which people are not clear. What it means to be equitable also needs much more careful analysis than it typically gets—geographical, social class, special needs for special groups, access, etc. Some people simply do not care about equity at all. And finally, the best institutional or environmental framework for accomplishing these objectives, even if we could agree what they were, is far from clear.

We are having a new institutional framework that I have previously advocated as an interesting one with which to experiment, but there is nothing in economics that tells us it is necessarily the right way. It may be a useful way. But the best institutional framework is clearly something that is highly contentious and while there is lots of theory we have desperately little actual experience of the sorts of things we are going in for right now. Unfortunately, the theory tells us that the efficiency characteristics of competition hinge crucially on how truly competitive—or contestable—markets are in practice. I fear there will be too much feather-bedding and over-regulation that substantially destroys local initiative while protecting what should not be protected.

I would echo Dr Cunningham and Sir Raymond this morning, in calling for a much greater emphasis on effectiveness to demonstrate beyond reasonable doubt that the productivity curve has really shifted up. That will at least remove one excuse for under-funding the health service, if you believe, as I do, that the balance of evidence does actually suggest that it is under-funded.

Even if the NHS does become more efficient in a more competitive and contestable market it will not necessarily be funded at the appropriate rate, but at least one excuse for under-funding will no longer exist. Ultimately the question of overall funding—in a system like ours and indeed in all systems that I am acquainted with in the world including the United States—is a political question. It is not a technical question and it is not for you or me to determine. Perhaps the worse we can hope for is to get the arguments much clearer in our heads and, I would hope as the years go by, much better evidence of what we actually get for our health dollars.

Chairman: Thank you very much indeed Tony.

9

Developing the purchaser role

MR ALASDAIR LIDDELL

Several speakers today have talked about the purchaser/provider split and I do not think many people here would argue with the proposition that the really radical feature of the Government's reforms is the creation of separate purchasers and providers. It is not surprising, in discussions about the White Paper, that this has led to a major focus on the new contractual relationship between districts and units.

What I would like to suggest is that contracting and purchasing will not be taking place in a vacuum; *what* is purchased will still be influenced by national and regional policy. *How* purchasing is undertaken—the contracting arrangements themselves—will require supervision to ensure that they work in the public interest.

Relatively little has been said or written about the region's role in relation to either of these factors. In East Anglia, we have been giving specific thought to influencing what is bought and in the time available today that is what I want to discuss. Our views are much less well formed on the regulatory role. All I can say is that there is a growing awareness amongst managers in my region—at regional, district, and unit level—that there is a need for one and that probably we will have it at the regional level.

The starting-point in considering what is bought is a recognition that the White Paper is about means and not ends. It provides us with some mechanisms the key aim of which—certainly in our region—is to ensure that the reforms are implemented to the benefit of the population that we serve. So if the White Paper is about means, it begs the question: 'What are our ends? What is it that we are trying to achieve?' I think it is necessary for us to be very clear about precisely what it is we are trying to do, say within a region, and how we organize ourselves to do it.

In East Anglia we spend around £500 million a year and employ through eight district health authorities about 35 000 staff. So the question is: to what purpose are these resources directed? We thought about that and without any pretence at originality came up with the following answer:

> 'Our purpose is to secure improvements in the health of the population of East Anglia by promoting health, preventing and diagnosing ill health, and ensuring the provision of appropriate health care and treatment for those suffering from illness or disability.'

We did think of asking the Department of Health what the mission of the NHS is, but concluded, 'No, don't let's do that; we might not like the answer!' So we worked out our own. The key words, for me, are 'our purpose is to secure improvements in health'. That is, in one sense, an obvious statement but it is also quite a radical statement. In the NHS we mostly respond to problems which people bring to us and which need to be solved. So, we are suggesting, the added value which we bring, or ought to bring with the use of public resources on a very large scale, is an improvement in health. Now there are of course many other factors and organizations which probably have a greater impact on the health of a population than we do. These include nutrition, housing, employment, and indeed the fiscal polices of Government itself. But in the NHS we have a unique contribution to make through health promotion, prevention, treatment, and care.

Table 7: Role of the RHA

- Planning—setting the strategic framework
- Resource allocation
- Performance review
- Managing change
- Providing some centralized services

If that is our purpose statement, what about our role at region in trying to fulfil that purpose? We came up with five elements (Table 7). For me probably the most important ones, apart from 'leading the process of change', are 'planning' and 'performance review'. 'Resource allocation' is allegedly going to get simpler. In any case, I think that should be subservient to what it is we are trying to achieve. It should reflect our plans and strategies. We do still provide some centralized services from region, although considerably fewer than a few months ago.

Table 8: Statement of values

- *Equity*—Equal treatment for equal need
- *Accessibility*—Geographic, time, language
- *Effectiveness*—In outcome terms
- *Efficiency*—Value for money
- *Appropriateness*—Relevance to need
- *Responsiveness*—To consumer wishes

The third element which we thought about and wanted to clarify was a statement of what our values are (Table 8). Again, not in any sense an original list, but one which we argued about and have become comfortable with in the end. We are demonstrating here that we are not just interested in financial performance, as perhaps commercial and industrial organizations are. In the public sector we are interested in providing benefits to the community which are not just financial benefits and this statement reflects the benefits which we are trying to provide. They are the criteria, if you like, for judging performance and this is certainly the sense in which we intend to use them within the region. Perhaps the most important of those is 'effectiveness' in outcome terms. Arguably, we should not be intervening in people's lives unless we have some confidence that we are going to be effective. The other elements, however, are important as well. This not to dismiss money as one underlying aspect of this, but looking also at responding to what consumers want out of the Health Service, in terms of access, equity and so on.

Of course, a statement like that just sounds rather like motherhood, apple pie, and pious hopes and usually is filed away. From our point of view, it is a rather important framework: it is a reference point for the decisions that we have to make. My Regional Health Authority has had a debate about breast cancer screening assessment and where it should be located in the region. This really revolved around quality and access, very explicitly using those terms and I think that is an entirely proper kind of debate for members of a health authority to have. It is nothing to do with operation of services—it is really the value judgements and the trade-off between the values which is important.

How are we going to apply this thinking in practice? I want to pick up on planning and performance review and talk a little bit about our thinking there.

First of all, what is wrong with our present approach to planning? I think we have made some progress in identifying health objectives, although frankly, not very much. Most of the money we spend in exactly the same way as it was spent last year. There is no direct link between NHS activity and the health of the population in our plans. There is a great assumption that the particular pattern of services and the way we deliver them is the best mix of responses which will achieve the best health result in terms of improving the health of the population. For the most part that is a gigantic and untested assumption. There is a focus on the margin: we are obsessed with the 2 per cent of savings, growth, or whatever it may be. The emphasis is on how we do things, not on what results we are trying to achieve. There is this complete obsession with financial performance—it is the only thing we can count and measure.

So if we are serious about improving the health of the population we need to identify the health improvements we are trying to achieve. We need to identify the areas where we can have some impact on the health of the population. We need to set ourselves some health objectives and to find some outcome measures which will tell us what progress we are making towards those objectives.

I want to illustrate this with sight as an aspect of health and ask you to imagine that you are in charge of improving the sight of the population within a region. How would you approach that and what sort of strategy would you develop for trying to achieve that aim? I suggest you might think about the groups of people who you would target in terms of those people who were already blind, those at risk of eye injury, those at risk of disease which might affect their sight, and those who were getting old. You might develop some actions to deal with improving the sight of those various groups which you could categorize under preventative actions, treatment, and continuing care (Table 9). You would then say, 'Let's devise some measures which will tell us whether we are being effective in improving sight' and you also might say, 'Let's keep a record of the number of people who are blind; let's think about how long it takes to get people who have eye injuries back into the community.' At the level of populations you could collect and monitor information which might give you an indication of the progress that you were making.

Table 9. Measures of health outcome effectiveness for 'sight' in a region

Sight	Prevention	Treatment	Continuing Care
Incapacity (Blindness)	HEALTH OUTCOME MEASURES		
Injury			
Disease			
Degeneration			

We are not just interested in effectiveness and health outcome. We are also interested in the other values that I put up earlier: access, equity, efficiency, appropriateness, and responsiveness. In a sense, the measures of quality that we are trying to achieve, and value for money. Again, you could find outcome measures. In the internal market, which conjures up the image of bussing people across the countryside for health care, you might particularly want to say under the heading of access: 'Well maybe no more than 15 per cent of people requiring in-patient treatment should have to travel more than 20 miles from where they live.' You could change the numbers according to what part of the country you were operating in and its specific problems. That would be a good outcome measure of access. You could come up with measures of waiting time and could think of other outcome measures.

In one sense, it is quite easy to talk about this at a conceptual level and for me it is perfectly obvious. In fact these are basic management principles: being clear about what you want to achieve and measuring your progress towards it. Of course, it is fundamentally difficult to do, in the context of health, otherwise lots of people would have done it long ago. What I would like to suggest is that it is possible, as well as right, to begin to make some progress in this direction. I know that many outcomes are separated from the intervention, often by many years, and for much of the time we do not even know what outcomes to expect from specific interventions. It does make you ask some penetrating questions when you begin to think in this way, and maybe it might prompt some of that research that one of the earlier speakers was talking about. Given that we do spend £26 billion on health care in this country, is it not time we asked some critical questions about what are the benefits of this input?

I think the advantages of this approach are that it establishes, or could establish over time, a much more direct link between NHS activities, say within a region, and the health of the population. That it starts from the patient's point of view by thinking what aspects of health—sight, mobility, reproduction, whatever it is—you are trying to improve and getting you to focus on those aspects that you can have some impact on through the use of the resources which are available to us in the Health Service. It gives us measures of benefit—a bottom line, if you like—that managers in industry take for granted. One which is not just expressed in terms of financial performance but health, quality, and value for money in general. It helps us think about the use of resources, not in an *ad hoc* way which reflects the historical accident of how the Health Service has grown up but in a more systematic way. Of course, it helps us to argue for more where there is a case for that.

How might this work in practice? Essentially, I see it as the region's role to negotiate with districts—the purchasing or commissioning agencies—the outcome measures that they plan to achieve during a specific period of planning. I use the word negotiation deliberately because I think that this process represents, as other speakers have pointed out, a rationing system (Table 10). Discretion operates by trading off some of these values: quality, cost, and access. You cannot have everything and there need to be some trade-offs. I think it is important that the actual trade-offs that are made reflect local perceptions about the needs of the local population. Similarly, you could trade-off in terms of different emphases on different aspects of health. This again should reflect local perceptions of what is appropriate for the population. So our job is to negotiate and make explicit the choices that have to be made—which, if you like, are rationing choices. These then become the targets to which the District Health Authority is working. The DHA then devises a service response in order to achieve these outcomes, balancing its judgement about the relative use of prevention, treatment, and care, and the different kinds of service responses which are available. That then forms the basis of its contracts.

Table 10. Measures of health outcome
- **Effectiveness**
- **Quality**
- **Value for money**

Sight	Prevention	Treatment	Care	Equity	Access	Efficiency	Appropriate	Responsive
Incapacity								
Injury								
Disease								
Degeneration								

I think this is a long-term project we have embarked upon, to put it mildly. We are at a very early stage of our thinking, and certainly we cannot hope to get health outcomes in this sense incorporated into the first round of contracts. We are, however, absolutely determined to avoid the first round of contracts being simply about money and volume. We have already started to talk with District Health Authorities, who support this approach, about how we can get health and quality into the decisions they make about the contracts they want to let for 1991 using this outcome basis. This will apply particularly in the area of quality, where it is rather easier to find measurable outcomes than initially in health. But we have also taken a longer term view about how we can produce health outcomes. We have two areas of work going on where groups of people are trying to produce worked examples based on sight and reproductive medicine. The reproductive medicine work in Norwich started with perinatal mortality as one of the most obvious outcome measures we have got. It brought together a group of health professionals who were engaged in this area of health. They are now thinking about what outcomes they are working to, recognizing that many of them have simply not been systematically measured in the past. I am very pleased to say there is a degree of enthusiasm about that. Indeed, the professionals involved thought it remarkable that despite their common purpose, this was the first time such a group had met.

The reproductive medicine group have attempted to define the scope of reproductive medicine as a starting-point. They decided that it covers from the onset of puberty through life to successful birth and survival through early childhood; a range from nine years of age for the parents to age seven of their child. This, I must say, left me wondering about the 24 months that they had not accounted for! In the same way, we are trying to develop a worked example in relation to 'sight' in Cambridge.

So, a beginning in tackling the longer-term question of how we can develop health and quality outcomes has been made, but is also touched with a practical approach which tries to get contracting off on the right foot.

In summary, what I am saying is whatever you may think about the White Paper—the time-scale, the ideology—the opportunities are there, if you are prepared to take them, to turn these reforms to our advantage, or more particularly to the advantage of the people who live in your particular locality.

Chairman: Thank you very much indeed.

10

Meeting the needs of the most vulnerable

PROFESSOR ELAINE MURPHY

I consider myself a rather fortunate, if peculiar, general manager, in that I was attracted to the job for the very reason that the Government was committed to certain changes in the Health Service. I think these changes have moved us further down a route which we had pioneered in Lewisham and North Southwark in a modest developmental way. These changes are characterized by major devolution of management to our units and attempting to set business programmes and service agreements which have been developing over the last two to three years.

I also happened to be in post when my own special clinical interest of community care has finally got onto the political agenda. The opportunities for improving care for chronically disabled and handicapped people have never been better, although I think it is just as well because they could scarcely get worse.

I am going to assume for the purposes of this talk, that when we talk of meeting the needs of the most vulnerable, we are talking largely about children with multiple handicaps, elderly people with chronic disabilities, physically or mentally handicapped people, and people with long-term mental illness. Those are the people who traditionally have received poor services and for whom many of us aspire to provide better services. They rarely figure in the media attention focused on the NHS and have very little consumer clout in the news. They do consume well over a third of our hospital resources and a much higher proportion of our primary care resources. They are the bulk users of our services.

Table 11. Expenditure by programme as percentage of NHS budget
(Source: Public Expenditure on Social Services)

	1970–71	*1984–85*
Primary care	19·3%	23·0%
General acute hospital/maternity	44·1%	36·8%
Elderly & physically handicapped	12·4%	16·6%
Mentally handicapped	4·1%	5·2%
Mentally ill	8·5%	7·9%
Children	7·1%	5·7%
Other	4·5%	8·0%

Table 11 shows the expenditure by programme in the NHS and shows how much it has shifted from 1971 to 1985. It does not identify very clearly all those groups individually, but you can see the general shift towards priority care and primary services. Please note the mental illness services, because they are the one service in so-called priority care services which managed to lose resources over this period of time.

The White Paper, however, was couched in the language of elective surgery. This has inevitably led to massive misunderstanding and resentment about the White Paper amongst clinicians involved in the priority care and vulnerable groups. I recently spoke to a joint meeting of the Royal College of Psychiatrists and the British Geriatric Society—300 or so psychiatrists and geriatricians. They were antipathetic to the ideas behind the White Paper and seemed convinced that nobody would want to purchase their services. There was a total lack of understanding about what the White Paper was intended to achieve. I think it a very sad reflection on the Government's communications exercise that we have so misled clinicians and made them fearful of what the White Paper might hold.

For the protection of vulnerable groups there are four areas which I think are important: (1) the strength and vision of a commissioning health authority; (2) the success of intersectoral planning to develop joint strategies; (3) proper funding and organization of community care; and (4) appropriate use of 'designated' or 'core' services in areas which will be dominated by large trusts.

The key to ensuring that services develop in an appropriate fashion is to keep in one's mind the needs of these individuals. Characteristically, their clinical needs are enormously diverse. The only thing these groups have in common is their dependence on others for help with the activities of daily life. Their common need is a social, not a clinical one. They also tend to need recurrent admissions to hospitals for what I would call the '10 000 mile service'. Crises need rapid response, rapid admission, and complex arrangements for discharge. I think too, that hospitals should feel like an integrated outreach from the community services and not vice versa. It is achieving these sorts of arrangements which I think are going to be essential for protecting these groups.

Let me come first to the strength of the commissioning authority. Surely separating hospitals from their purchasing authorities will lead to a concentration of effort by authorities in discovering what it is that the local community want, as well as what the public health data tell us we need. An authority must, however, have buying clout if we are not to become dominated by one monopolistic local provider (Table 12). If the large teaching hospitals or large district general hospitals, that have traditionally dominated health care, are allowed to become more dominant than the commissioning authority, we will lose flexibility. We will have less ability to take risks and be less able to respond creatively in ways that local people want.

A health authority in the future really only has to ask itself four questions. What kinds of health services do we need? Who can we buy them from? How do we know we are getting value for money? How do we know that it is working in terms of the public health strategy for the local population? It is this last question, I believe, which can protect the most vulnerable. Health authorities' actions, of course, must provide answers to these questions.

For this last question, 'Developing a strategy: how do we know it is working for the population?', the answer must be to develop a communication and information strategy about what is going on out there. Getting close to the population and listening to how they feel is more likely to protect vulnerable groups than any amount of designation of core services. The pressure groups that people should be communicating with are often more concerned about the bread and butter services than they are with the one-off or local high-tech services. The Community Health Council's concerns are nearly always about the problems of the ordinary and the long-term patients. I see all the complaints that come from Members of Parliament in my district and I assure you that the vast majority of them, both from the CHC and from MPs, are about the vulnerable groups.

Obviously, we need to get close to GPs, patients, and local authorities and to do market research of the local population. It must be a two-way education as well as receiving information. At the moment we do not do this at all. We simply do not take seriously the views of anyone out there, nor do we employ communication and information specialists. We employ information data analysts and information technology people, who of course provide valuable skills which we must have; but we have never employed anybody to really find out what is happening out there. I think that this is one way that we will be able to protect the vulnerable.

Table 12. Criteria for a commissioning authority

- Buying power
- Manpower and management capability
- Workable geography
- Uniform social demography
- Manageable numbers of contracts
- Coterminosity with FPC
- Coterminosity with local authority
- Diversity and quality of teaching

A last point on the theme of developing a strong, effective commissioning health authority, is my criteria for how you can make it strong and effective. It must have buying power and clout to prevent the domination by providers. It simply must have the management capability to negotiate with very tough clinicians and managers. It helps if the geography is right. If the social demography is fairly uniform it makes planning a lot easier. It must have as few contracts to manage as possible if it is going to be effective. And, of course, it should be coterminous with the FPC and should be able to provide coterminosity for planning of community care with the local authority. Finally, it should provide a diversity and quality of teaching if we are to foster the kinds of quality of service and calibre of people who will be interested in continuing to provide a Health Service for the vulnerable groups (Table 12).

Let me return to my other themes. My second protection for the vulnerable groups is the strength of inter-sectoral relationships with the FPC, GPs, and local authorities. I have in the past, as a general manager, been so consumed by operational management matters that 'foreign policies' had to take a back seat. I genuinely believe that in the future, without those direct management responsibilities and the emphasis on developing a health care strategy, that I shall have far greater time to develop closer links with my opposite numbers at the FPC and local authorities.

The third area, of course, is the proper funding and organization of community care. The two White Papers I think must be seen in conjunction and implemented as a single new approach. 'Griffiths II', or *Caring for People*—as its banal name is—and *Working for Patients* are strikingly similar in many ways (Table 13).

Table 13: Similarities between *Working for Patients* and *Caring for People*

1. Separation of service design and purchase from provision function.
2. Management of services by contract.
3. Mixed economy of care.
4. Development of information systems for case management and costing.
5. Cultural shift towards accountability.

The separation of buying and providing roles, the management of services by contract, developing mixed economy of care, the development of information systems on which we will be dependent to do the management, and the cultural shift in both authorities to more explicit accountability—these common features should enable health and local authorities to develop common philosophies about the style of delivery of service for priority care groups.

They also highlight, I think, the relative infancy of both health and local authorities in certain key areas. The advantages of co-operation between authorities to share necessary skills and resources, particularly in developing information systems for work in the community, are obvious. But Government's relationship with the local authority is very different from that with health authorities. While *Working for Patients* contained a lot of directives, *Caring for People* is couched in the language of persuasion. As a consequence it sadly falls into what Roy Griffiths himself called 'the discredited refuge of exhortation to joint planning'. While the White Paper acknowledges that current joint planning processes have failed miserably, we get three pages on so-called 'collaborative working' ending with the lame statement that 'further consideration will be given'. Having had contact with the Department since then on where they have got to on their further considerations, I can tell you they have not got very far yet. This probably means that you and I will have to work out how to implement *Caring for People* just as we go along, as we do for *Working for Patients*.

The other mystifying area is the new trench which is to be dug between health care and social care. If health care is diagnosis, treatment, and rehabilitation, and social care is the supported activities of daily life, why is it that in *Caring for People*, health authorities may carry on providing long-stay care for disabled, elderly, and others and remain the registering body for private and voluntary nursing homes?

The populations in long-term hospital and nursing care are largely in receipt of social care and should receive health care only as required by each individual. It seems to me that the present proposals for community care could leave the health authorities isolated and hospital-bound, still consuming massive resources over which the local authorities will have almost no influence. While *Caring for People* proposals give the usual exhortation, as I say, to joint planning, I cannot see how this is to be achieved except in the case of discharged mental hospital patients. Nevertheless, obviously we have to try as far as we can.

This session is supposed to be about developing a seamless service. Professionals who work in the fields of these groups do talk endlessly about developing the seamless service. By this they usually mean an integrated, comprehensive service across acute hospital beds, community provision of hostels, domiciliary services in people's own homes, and one team running a whole service. It usually means one telephone number, with a bit of luck! In practice, this is rarely achieved in conjunction with local authorities and almost never includes the private and voluntary sectors. Nevertheless, it is what most people aspire to. Certainly the separation of health care from social care is extremely difficult in practice, particularly where in treating a disorder, for example a severe depression or a physical condition such as Parkinson's Disease, response to treatment is sometimes best monitored by noting an individual's progress in managing the tasks of daily life. It seems to me that it is crucial that future proposals cement existing service integration as well as fostering much closer working between health and local authority personnel than we have at the moment.

Figure 10 represents my understanding of the Community Care White Paper, with the separation of the two sectors; the integration that we seek can be achieved in two ways. One is by joining up the provider services across sectors. There are at the moment quite a number of successful ventures in almost all districts, often started up with joint funding and providing health care and social care in one unit or providing a joint community care service. But such joint ventures will not ensure that a district has a common strategic plan. I think the solution to this could be a radical but simple one: that the two statutory authorities could form a joint buying consortium.

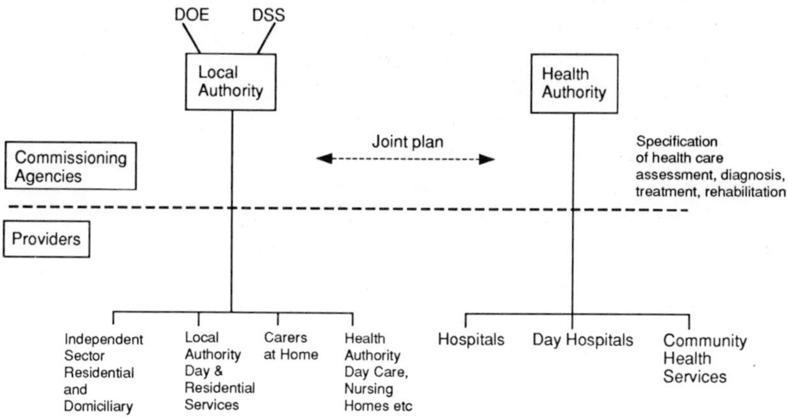

Fig. 10. Griffiths II Government proposals.

A new organization which could be pooling the health service priority care revenue and the local authority social service resources for domiciliary, residential, and day-care services. I do think the local authority must be the key agency around which services are developed. Obviously, to make these links, we do need a coterminosity of organizations.

Figure 11 represents what my joint buying consortium would look like. Now there are obvious drawbacks to this proposal and it will not surprise you to learn that where I come from in Southwark this plan has not met locally with universal acclaim. I believe that where it is politically possible it is the best solution. The alternative is to stagger on towards a joint strategic plan but with no real integration or a common approach.

My last way of protecting the vulnerable groups is by designating a service as a core service—I believe the phrase is going to be now 'a designated service'. I think the Department of Health must rue the day when they introduced this concept as it has been interpreted in so many ways in different places.

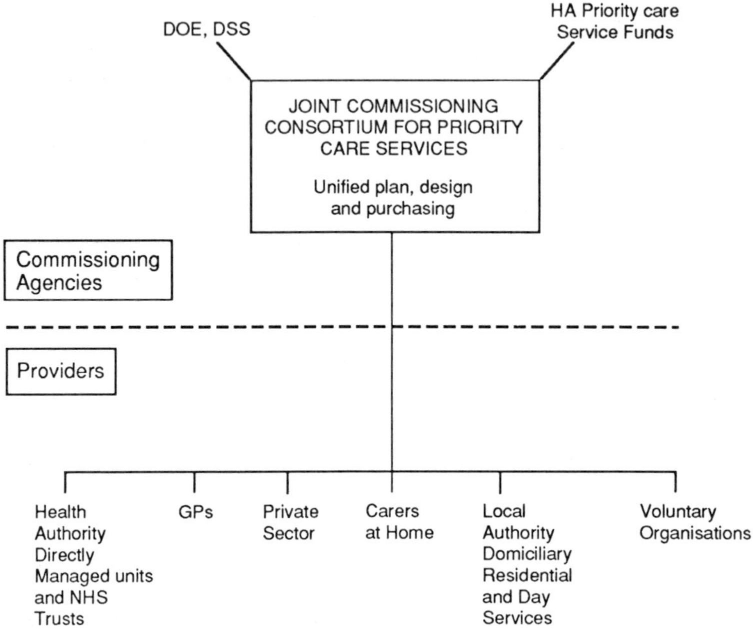

Fig. 11. Proposals for a community care consortium buying agency.

The concept, of course, is only necessary for services bought from a monopoly providing self-governing trust, when the trust is the only provider or is indeed an essential part of a local service. Perhaps the only thing we need to take note of is what is required for guaranteed local access. Health authorities will need to define these services in terms of the need for accessibility. I think accessibility depends on a number of factors:

1. characteristics of the local population: income, education, social deprivation.
2. characteristics of local health care provision: quantity, quality, physical accessibility.
3. use of current services.
4. indices of travel: transport time, delays, etc.
5. satisfaction with local services.

One needs to take into account whether or not people do need the services locally. This is very much a judgement that needs to be made very differently in authorities around the country. What is right for Alasdair Liddell's North Suffolk, or wherever, will be very different from Lewisham and North Southwark.

In practice, particularly in towns and suburban areas, it is likely that only those services which are currently organized in catchment areas will need to be designated in the first place as core services. After all, catchment areas were designed to cope with the very anxieties that core services are designed to address. You do not want anybody falling outside the net of somebody having responsibility.

If we add to that all the emergency admissions that come through a casualty or accident and emergency department, you actually add up to 75 per cent of the work of any large hospital. It seems highly unlikely that trusts will want to jeopardize or give up these particular services. Basically they constitute the bed-rock income as well as the bed-rock of services for teaching medical undergraduates, junior doctors, and other professionals. Out of town it may be more important to designate other services as core services.

Finally, how we can ensure that there is no two-tier system that leaves the vulnerable groups dependent on a second-rate, directly managed service and leaves the glamorous trusts to go their own route? It seems to me that the only possible way of avoiding this—and I believe it is a really dangerous spectre that we should avoid—is to ensure that everybody becomes separated off as a trust as soon as possible. That we construct a system whereby the health authorities can genuinely concentrate on developing their commissioning role, forget their provider role and make sure that the trusts cover the full range of community and hospital services. These need not necessarily be in the same trust because the co-ordinating role can be at centre. I think this is far safer than that we have a handful of glamorous trusts established in the first year and that we then end up with a two-tier system where nobody will be satisfied.

11

Discussion

Dr Peter Sheridan: It seems to me that, as a GP I am going to have one role in *Working for Patients*, where I will be encouraged to audit and act as a gatekeeper to hospital services, whilst in terms of *Caring for People* I am the patient's advocate. I wonder whether Professor Murphy would like to comment on whether the independent contractor status would be important for patient's advocates within the Health and Social Services. Would she also like to comment on whether she thinks that a service where social services departments and health authorities are coterminous and joined together as buying authorities, is in fact seamless, if the FPC is left on the edge?

Professor Elaine Murphy: I think you have made a number of interesting points. I must confess I had not seen the role of general practitioners quite that way before. I think you are not the only ones who will face that dual role; the new case managers in local authorities will have exactly the same problem. Indeed there is a theme, which goes through a lot of the case management literature, of responsibility for a budget and gatekeeping, together with responsibility to act as an advocate. It is a difficult issue but there is a lot you can read about it.

As I only had limited time, I missed out what I believe is absolutely fundamental. The trust that is being developed at Guys, Lewisham and the mental illness services in Lewisham and North Southwark deliberately omits the community health services, because the community trust should be developed in conjunction with the FPC and LMC. The sooner that we can marry them together, which is obviously politically and legally not feasible at the moment, and the sooner we can develop the community health services as a contractor which looks mainly to the FPC, then the easier it will be.

Dr Peter Jaffe: Many departments have spent ten years or more trying to create the links with those community services which, it seems to me, you are saying should now be split. Do you then feel that there is no place for a system in which the hospital and the community sections of a particular service are actually integrated into the same organization?

Professor Elaine Murphy: I think the issue is that we must be very clear about what role a community outreach service is playing. Most of the community health services relate to primary care and prevention services and their natural home is clearly with general practice. I have personally been a great advocate for developing community outreach services from the hospitals. There are some secondary and tertiary services which it seems very sensible to provide as outreach from the hospitals. They could therefore just as easily be provided managerially from the hospital end. This does not mean to say that hospital-managed people have to remain within the hospital walls. What I think we must be very careful to enable is the development of knowledge and expertise in general practice in regard to certain diagnoses. I am for example thinking here of diabetes and certain rheumatological conditions. Shared care for these conditions requires an intense commitment from the general practitioner such that the outreach services might not develop optimally from the hospital base. Though I would not discourage them I am only saying this has to be done in a sensitive way in conjunction with GPs. I do not think it matters where they are managed from.

Dr John Gabbay: Alasdair Liddell put up a very nice model of methods of attaining measures in health outcome. I wonder whether he has sufficient experience to know how much resource would be required to go through that matrix for each parameter.

Mr Alasdair Liddell: I think there is a great danger of turning that kind of exercise into a huge paper-chase. In a sense one can visualize my matrix as being an endless spreadsheet—for those of you who are computer-literate—which goes off the screen in every direction. It would be completely fruitless if that actually happened. Firstly, you have to think about where you are in the organization; secondly you have to think about priorities and impact. At regional level we will be looking at the performance of a District Health Authority. We will look at populations and take a fairly broad-brush view of outcome measures which we will want to identify and track as part of our performance review or monitoring process. To begin with we will select the easier kinds of outcomes, those that are more easily measured, and see how we get on with them. We will also select those areas where we think there might be a need to get people to rethink the current pattern of service provision or where we could have maximum short-term impact. So one begins to build up—you don't try and do it all at once. Ultimately, you are selecting from potentially millions of possible outcome measures and you need to identify outcome measures that you want to follow and track. All of this is really about encouraging a new way of thinking or a new set of attitudes to what it is we are trying to do. We have a little label on our letterhead—'Managing Better Health'. This is to remind everybody who works in the region of the basic notion of what it is that we are trying to do.

Certainly I think that to develop the sort of ideas I was talking about to the full would require resources. A certain amount of management resource in terms of collecting and analysing the information, and quite a lot of resource in terms of managerially driven research to supplement the research that is already going on.

Professor Tony Culyer: I agree with Alasdair. I think it is terribly important, in all this talk about mission, objectives, and outcome measurement not to permit the perfect to become the enemy of the merely good. These measures are not substitutes for the exercise of judgement: they are aids to judgement. How far you go along with the development of sophisticated techniques or measures is a question of judgement and has to be made at the local level. Just as it is a question of judgement how much research you want to put into the development of methodologies. Similarly it is a question of judgement about how many resources you want to put into things like information technology. Do not forget, capitalism has operated a price mechanism, of the sort that we are now developing in the Health Service, without information technology. Private markets do not necessarily depend upon the existence of sophisticated outcome measures. They do not necessarily depend for their efficient functioning on very sophisticated accounting systems. These may help, but it is again a question of judgement about what is the optimal degree of resource deployment to all of these various activities, whether they be information systems, outcome measures or research activities and so on. It is always a question of judgement.

Dr Jim Connelly: Could the panel talk about the perverse incentives that we have heard about. There are two types of budgets: there is a health care budget and there is a social care budget. First, who defines what is health care and who defines what is social care? Second, if there are disputes, who will suffer?

Professor Elaine Murphy: I think that this is the major problem that has not been solved by the Community Care White Paper, particularly in relation to elderly people. I think there will be enormous incentives to shuffle severely disabled elderly people backwards and forwards across health and social services. It is this very fear that drives me at least to try to get some agreement on a strategic plan to define the degrees of dependency of people when they will become the responsibility of health and social services. I think there is considerable fear at the moment that we will all be shuffling it off to the neighbour down the road: I see nothing that will actually make that any better at the moment.

Mr Alasdair Liddell: There was a certain amount of speculation this morning as to the motives behind the White Paper and what was in people's minds. Now that is always entertaining to talk about. My own view is that this is not the only flaw in the logic. There are others that will become apparent. I think one of the great virtues of the White Paper is that it is in fact so vague about precisely how all this will work in practice. Correspondingly I think that is why it is so important that those of us in the Health Service actually seize the initiative, that we identify the weak links and then start thinking about how we are going to make them work. I have heard all the arguments about why there should not be pilots and experiments from the Government. I very strongly believe that there should be what we call 'development work' in East Anglia, because that is the way we get money out of the Department. If we call them 'pilots' or 'experiments' we do not get money out of the Department. I think it is very important that instead of intellectualizing about these problems, we actually get in there and experience them as soon as possible so that we can figure out ways round them. I do not have a particular answer to that specific perverse incentive, which I agree exists, but there are others in the system which need to be identified and tackled.

Professor Tony Culyer: There is another area of incentives I might just touch on. Although some of these things are undoubtedly vague at the moment, some of them are going to become very precise in the not too distant future. I think it is highly likely to become true in the pricing area. First, as I guess most of you will know, the Department of Health is extremely exercised about the dangers of monopoly practices, especially coupled with the dangers of there being insufficient incentives for purchasing authorities to seek out multiple bidders for contracts. In either of those contexts they have yet to determine whether or not they are going to go for a rather dirigiste approach by having, either a central price schedule, perhaps by DRG—which I personally think would be a disaster, or a modified version in which a centrally promulgated pricing rule will have to be adopted by providers. Secondly, they could leave it much more to local discretion. This would rely on simple openness in costing or pricing, or on competition for franchises of local provider units. There are a whole lot of possibilities there that are still very actively under discussion. This is an area which is going to have huge implications for the incentive structures, especially within the health sector.

Dr Nick Black: The one encouraging observation I have made today is a general acceptance of the importance of outcomes and the effectiveness of health services. Virtually every speaker has acknowledged that. Nobody has identified, though, how we are going to increase our knowledge of outcome. Who is actually going to fund the vast research effort that is required? I would be particularly interested in the managers' views on this, because, on the whole, the NHS record of funding research and development has been appalling. That is probably understating it when one looks at the actual percentage. No other organization in any other sector would have survived on the under-funding of research and development.

Professor Margaret Turner-Warwick: Would you allow me to add my question to this because it is almost identical?

Looking at Mr Liddell's matrix I was having just the same thoughts. You could analyse his health outcomes in terms of health service and biomedical research. They have been around a very long time and the problems have also been around a long time. You will remember when Rothschild took a third of the Medical Research Council's money back to the Department of Health in order to give health services research an attempted boost. This was unsuccessful for a whole number of complex reasons. To think that these are issues that have been invented with the White Paper for the first time is incorrect.

My question is linked with the previous one. Does the panel believe that the new Chief Research and Development Adviser will be able to entrap the money that we have so long been seeking for both biomedical and health services research?

Mr Alasdair Liddell: I do not know what will happen nationally; perhaps not surprisingly, my focus is a regional one. I do not know whether the ideas that we have been talking about in East Anglia will be picked up by other regions and run nationally. There may be more emphasis on research from a national level, but I think if we are going to achieve our objectives we have to recognize that we will have to fund that from the resources that are available within our region. I imagine that most of the impetus for that will come from us at the RHA and those in purchasing authorities, whose role is to assess the health of the population and find ways of meeting that need. Why should it be any different from the past? I am not pretending that any of the ideas I have talked about are new. There are different conditions. I think the focusing of roles at region, district, and unit level, which the White Paper has brought, is helpful in focusing our attention on what is essential. My view is that increasingly, both within the managerial as well as the professional hierarchies, we have come to appreciate the importance of outcome. We will be willing and will need to find answers to questions which have remained unanswered. I think the combined managerial and health professionals' thirst for knowledge might have some impact on our record of investment.

Professor Margaret Turner-Warwick: One point of clarification. I do not believe that the role of the Chief Research and Development Adviser will be to conduct centralized research, but rather to see that the job is done, presumably by the regions, districts, or universities. I indeed hope a little might come the College way. They will be conducting the whole operation to ensure that it is done better than in the past. It has failed in the past through lack of resources and I wondered whether you had any more confidence in the availability of resources in the future?

Mr Alasdair Liddell: In a nutshell—I personally do have confidence. I do not know whether we will get extra resources. I think we will have to make some hard choices about the way we use our existing resources. Do we go on blindly putting all our money into the existing patterns of service? Or do we try and question whether there are more appropriate ways of actually spending that money and be prepared to invest a little to find out the answer to that question? I am optimistic.

Professor Elaine Murphy: Well I'm glad Alasdair is optimistic. As you said, who is going to fund it and who is going to do it? I would turn the question back to Dr Black and Professor Holland and say I hope they are going to do it.

Who is going to fund it? I see it as an absolutely fundamental role for the regions. Any large organization which is in the business of manufacturing would normally expect to spend 1–2 per cent of its annual revenue or turnover on research and development. That means in South East Thames, for example, out of their £1 billion per year we would be expecting them to spend £10–20 million per year on research.

I honestly think that, unless regions take the bull by the horns and decide that they will be the key research and development funders for their populations, then I really do not see anybody else doing it. I think it is unlikely to happen centrally because it requires a drive of the kind that exists at regional level. I think they are the people who should fund it.

Professor Tony Culyer: A comment and a suggestion. The comment is that the reason why it didn't happen in the past is entirely because of clinical capture of the research budget. The suggestion is that I suspect a vast majority of you here are members of the Institute of Health Service Management. I suggest you use that in order to bring appropriate weight to bear at region or other appropriate places.

Dr M. Impallomeni: Health is directly proportional to income, and the poor are those whose health is more at risk. If that is the case, I wonder whether in fact poverty—which is one of the characteristics of many elderly people and one of the factors which makes them vulnerable—is something which is not really addressed in the White Paper.

Secondly, I would like to ask Professor Murphy whether she is convinced that both White Papers are really for the improvement of the care of elderly people—both health and social care? What evidence is available which makes this clear to her? I wonder whether she knows that long-stay wards are already being offered to private enterprise up and down the country and whether she really believes that this is the result of the planned improvement of services for the care of the elderly, or the result of under-financing of health services?

Professor Tony Culyer: There is a very high correlation between the ill-health experience of people and the lowness of their incomes. This incidentally has a rather interesting implication for the discussion of equity and efficiency. In the vast majority of cases the biggest health improvement is to be had amongst the poorer and more deprived members of the community, so that, to a large extent, an equitable concern forces resources in much the same way as an efficiency concern. Sometimes those things are presented as if they were in conflict, but I think in large part in our health care system that is not the case.

Professor Elaine Murphy: I think we have to acknowledge now that over 50 per cent of long-stay care for the elderly is provided by the private sector, whether we like it or not. It has happened in a totally unplanned *ad hoc* fashion. The only hope I have for the future is that at least there will be some definite strategic decision to use private care as opposed to health service care. In that sense I think there is a chance that it will be better planned and used. If you ask me if I am confident that things will necessarily improve, then I am not.

Dr M. Impallomeni: My question was—what evidence is there that the planning will bring about an improvement in the care of the elderly?

Professor Elaine Murphy: I do not think we have any evidence right now that it will.

Professor Lou Opit: Can I just make a comment and then ask a question? The comment is that I am afraid that the overwhelming rhetoric and the flavour of the month 'quality of outcome' is something which I do not share, given that many of the outcomes in medical services are social goals which are immensely complicated to measure and to interpret. There has been an assumption that, if you had the information, somehow you were able to move forward, but many of the problems are actually interpretative, both philosophical and technical.

What I want to know is: what does equal treatment for equal need actually mean? It doesn't mean anything to me. And: why wasn't it equal treatment based on equal outcome?

Professor Tony Culyer: I am not sure what 'equal treatment for equal needs' means either. There are huge logical and philosophical differences. Not least the word 'need' which needs to be followed by a preposition: 'need for...' what? This gets you right into Lou's sort of territory whereby you cannot really separate the demand and the supply side because a need is going to be conditional either upon what you have or what you imagine you might eventually have. It is a very complex thing.

However, I would thoroughly support the discussion of 'need', 'outcome', 'equity', and so on. It helps people to think about what are immensely important and difficult issues. There are no final solutions and nobody pretends there are, but at least we can try to structure our thinking.

Chairman: I think that this afternoon has clearly demonstrated some of the problems and I am extremely grateful to the three speakers for such stimulating presentations.

I think I would just like to just emphasize three points that came out in both the talks and the discussion. I am delighted, as a public health practitioner, that the two non-medical members of the panel were concerned with changing and improving health status as their definition of what they were trying to achieve. I have some pessimism about what Professor Murphy said about changing budgets. It was interesting that the major area of diminution in expenditure over the time period 1971–84 was in mental illness, so that her optimism is, perhaps, a little bit tainted. And finally, I think it is worth commenting that only those in Academe have been concerned in the discussion on research within the Health Service. Elsewhere, there has been a deafening silence.

Session 3: Doctors and the new Health Service

DR JOHN MARKS—Chairman

I thought a session which was called 'Doctors and the new Health Service' would be a good time to read my favourite quotation from the White Paper. As it is hidden in the Scottish Section most of you have probably never seen it. It is paragraph 10(11): 'It is doctors not politicians or managers who treat patients...' and it goes on: '...and the Government is therefore seeking the full co-operation of the profession'. Now Kafka may be dead, but George Orwell is alive and kicking!

There are two intractable problems which have faced the Health Service since the first day it started. One is funding, and the other is medical manpower—which we have got wrong on at least four occasions.

12

Planning the numbers

DR ANGELA JONES

The White Paper proposes many changes in the health services. It seems to be giving new freedoms to encourage self-determination and competition and all those good things about the market place. But there appear to be no freedoms at all in medical manpower.

The Secretary of State remains committed to the principles of achieving a balance. What does this mean? It actually means in practice that all the existing controls that we face now will be retained. Now, will these controls also apply to the NHS trust hospitals? Although they have the novel freedom of being able to vary the pay and conditions of their staff, including medical staff, they must comply with the Government policy relating to the numbers of hours juniors work. They are also expected to follow the Government policy as set out in 'Achieving a Balance'. So no freedom here either for the darlings of the new era—the trust hospitals.

What are the controls which the profession and the Government are committed to, in spite of all the other major changes that are going on? These changes were set out in 'Achieving a Balance' and 'Plan for Action'. The proposals are for consultant expansion, which is in fact happening with the aim of improving patient care. The other aim is to get the senior registrars and registrars into balance, and to hold some control on the senior house officers. The idea is that by matching the number of doctors in training to the availability of consultant posts, junior doctors will have a greater chance than ever in the past of progression to a career post without an unnecessarily long time in training. That is the theory.

How are these controls worked out? There is the central committee, the joint planning advisory committee or JPAC as it is known. This determines, using the best evidence that is available, the likely future consultant numbers, taking into consideration the length of time people have to be in training, the numbers of senior registrars and career registrars for each specialty. It then allocates specialty-specific quotas to all the regions. Not an easy task and one fraught with dangers. Now registrars are particularly interesting as they are divided into career and visiting posts. The visiting posts are only available for doctors from overseas who will be returning to their own country and who cannot remain for a career in this country. The career registrars are people who are looking to obtain consultant posts in this country. This, by the way, also includes EEC doctors. Their numbers are controlled and relate to available consultant posts being based on retirements and any new developments. In addition, they are distributed to the regions using a formula which is one career post per acute specialty per district and weightings for population and teaching; this is to try to get some equity in distribution. It is in these career registrars where the greatest changes are seen. Especially in terms of service-load carried by these doctors in training, we are going to have to face major changes.

Table 14: Career registrar quotas in North West Thames Regional Health Authority

	Now	**Then**
General medicine	77	31
General surgery	51	19
Paediatrics	20	14
Trauma and orthopaedics	12	7
Anaesthetics	39	12
Obstetrics & gynaecology	19	11

Table 14 shows the indicative quotas for career posts in North West Thames: the actual quotas have not been issued yet. You can see some interesting reductions which have to be achieved over time. The figures should in fact be considered together with the visiting registrars because established posts which will not be required for career registrars can be filled by visiting registrars. So, for example if we look at general surgery, the difference between 19 and 51 posts can be made up by filling 32 posts with visiting registrars and the numbers could in fact stay the same.

However, it is not possible to say whether all the specialties in all the regions will be able to recruit their full quota of overseas registrars. If they cannot, the service will have to be covered in another way. Is there much flexibility for doing this? Currently, there is no move by the consultants to take over work done by juniors, so consultant expansion may not be the answer to this problem.

Is there another way? There are three other grades of staff who are not in training and so can be considered as service posts only. There is the new grade, the staff grade, but here again the numbers are controlled and limited to 10 per cent of consultant numbers. So I do not suppose they will be able to pick up all the service provision that may be needed when the numbers change. Then there are associate specialists, but these are personal posts and they cannot be advertised or openly recruited to. Finally, there is very limited help available from clinical assistants who can work up to only five sessions. It seems to me there is a need for a radical change in the traditional way that hospitals are staffed.

There is, in addition, another requirement: the safety net. With all the changes going on amongst the intermediate staff, especially for the acute services, in the hospitals it has been agreed that the number of intermediate staff should not go below a safe level to support consultants. The safety net has not in fact been defined and as you can imagine it varies between the specialties as well as between hospitals.

General medicine, general surgery, trauma and orthopaedics, obstetrics and gynaecology, paediatrics, and anaesthetics are the specialties where a safety net has to be provided. They must be adequately and safely staffed, however this is defined. Will the changes in the numbers and the controls on medical staff allow this? We have some preliminary answers. All regions were asked by the Department of Health to undergo a safety net review. The conclusions are that it may not be possible, in all specialties and in all hospitals, to provide a safety net given the likely changes in numbers.

As well as the safety net there is a real need to reduce the junior doctors' hours of work. We have to get to an average of 72 hours per week to reduce what is called 'onerous rotas'. What this really means, if you work it out at its simplest level, is that in order to achieve an average 72 hours per week for junior doctors you require four juniors to arrive at the right rota. This is unlikely to be achieved with the control on the numbers that we have, the lack of ability to mix the different grades and the inappropriateness of cross-specialty cover in many cases.

Again, if there is no change in the traditional way we do things, the way we staff hospitals, I do not know how we will manage the future.

Additionally, the junior doctors are doctors in training and the training requirements for the various specialties that the Colleges set out have to be considered. Some of these requirements do need revision because the practice of medicine has moved on and it does seem sometimes that approval is based on what used to happen and not what is actually happening now. Anyway, increasing or restricting the number of juniors either causes dilution of clinical experience or else puts too heavy a burden on them. In fact this playing around with the numbers can seriously affect educational recognition.

However, the White Paper provides an opportunity for improving the distribution and the training for juniors in a way that we did not have in the past. This is the idea of regional training contracts. If this is developed flexibly, with care and thought for what it is we are trying to do and how we are trying to do the training, we can improve and strengthen training even with the changes in numbers that are facing us.

What about the trust hospitals? Clearly they will want to be involved in contracting for training. They will have to keep within the numbers and they will have to take the reduction in junior hours seriously. But what about their freedom? This key freedom, I think, is interesting. It gives them the right to determine pay and conditions for the medical staff. This includes not only the consultants but also the medical staff in training. Will this mean that they will scoop the market for the reduced number of juniors? They might. Or will they look for a new style of consultant, one who is much more involved with direct patient care and give them pay and conditions that make this new way of working highly attractive and popular? If that happens, what will be the effect on the consultants not employed by these trusts? What effect will this have on the planning of consultant numbers and the planning of the junior numbers?

In considering all these things—the aims of 'Achieving a Balance', the safety net requirements, the need to reduce the junior doctors' hours, the training requirements—they all seem to be working against one another. It all seems incompatible. You also have to bear in mind that the juniors now provide essential emergency and routine front-line care and that has to continue. So are there any solutions? How can all of this be reconciled, particularly in the new NHS?

I would like to make some suggestions as to how it might be possible to satisfy all these conflicting requirements. What about reducing the number of sites on which acute specialties are provided? This would certainly ease the manpower problems, but it is very difficult to achieve and politically often unacceptable. It certainly takes a long time. Uneconomic and inefficient units may be rationalized to provide fewer, larger units. That certainly would help junior hours and training.

What about developing acute and cold hospitals? Hospitals could link together, some providing elective surgery and others covering the emergency work. You would not need full safety nets in both types of hospitals and training could be maintained by flexibility and suitable rotations that give the right range and experience. You could also have a single hospital with different staffing patterns in different specialties. For example, a hospital could staff its anaesthetic department with consultants only while the surgical department was more traditionally staffed with the usual tiers of juniors. Or should we in fact look to developing hospitals where juniors are trained with full safety nets and other hospitals that are run and staffed by consultants and non-training grades, such as the staff grade? Certainly if the restrictions on the staff grade were eased this would be possible. There may be more doctors out there than we realize who would be happy to work as staff grade in this sort of situation.

These are just a few suggestions. I think that all of these proposals must be explored and considered if the profession and the Government wish to hold to the agreements on medical manpower. I think that the White Paper gives us a chance to rethink the ways hospitals are staffed both by consultants and juniors. I also think that if we are careful and sensible about it, it will give us an opportunity to achieve a better structure and to improve training.

Finally, I cannot leave the question of doctor numbers and changes in patterns of work without referring to the consultants of the future. However the pattern of staffing will develop the nature of consultant work will change. I am sure that the average consultant in the new Health Service will spend maybe only 50 per cent of time on what might be called 'hands-on clinical activity', with a split in that clinical activity between routine general work and specialist work. This will depend on the type of hospital the person works in. But there is another whole area of, if you like, non-clinical work that will be developed. This includes the role as teacher, learner, manager, administrator, politician, and advocate as well as the important audit role. I think the role of politician and advocate in the new Health Service is one which every consultant will have to take seriously. The new role will also include teaching and learning new techniques. Every consultant may periodically have a year's sabbatical. What I think I am trying to say is that these non-clinical activities are important and they are legitimate. They are not done as optional extras but they are actually part of the consultant's work of the future.

Relating this back to numbers, it means that we have to consider these issues and plan the consultant numbers for the future, based on this type of pattern of work. I would also say that anyone who does not want to be involved with non-clinical activities does not want to be a consultant and they should do something else instead.

I think we must plan our consultant expansion and hope that we will, so that the numbers allow for first class and sufficient patient care and probably, as good measure, will also improve the management in the Health Service.

Chairman: Well, there is plenty of room for thought there and I suspect there will be some very interesting questions.

13

Medical education and research

PROFESSOR MARGARET TURNER-WARWICK

'Misunderstanding' in the White Paper is a famous phrase. I think there is a lot of misunderstanding about what education and the full scope of research are really about. First, I must say something about doctoring. I think most doctors actually love change. You only have to look at many general practitioners and consultants trying to use the most modern drugs even when their therapeutic use are not finally agreed upon. The tendency is to try to keep up with the changes in medicine, not the reverse. Of course, in good doctoring, this enthusiasm for the latest ideas has to be tempered with rigorous self-discipline and responsibility so that we do not go too far, too fast, and find that innovations have not been adequately tested or justified to ensure that they provide at least some element of good for the patients. Because of the White Paper and the instability that it has created, there is a tendency amongst some almost to believe that medicine has never been practised before! The Hippocratic Oath does go back about 2500 years reflecting the medical ethos of doctors being primarily responsible for the care and the welfare of their patients. The idea that doctoring is something apart from this responsibility is totally strange to me. I think we really have to correct this balance.

This College, dare I say, has been about medical standards for 472 years. We have had the capacity, for instance, to inspect the Apothecaries to ensure that they were not prescribing compounds which we thought had not been adequately tested in medicine. This has gone on for several centuries. I am not looking back or being a fuddy-duddy. Medicine is about caring for patients and scrutinizing new therapies, ensuring that what we do in the future is no worse than what we did before. This is something that has taken place over a very long period of time, which I think we need to bear in mind. I passionately believe that good doctoring is about the care of the individual patient as well as populations. We must not lose sight of that.

Education and research in medicine concerns not only the statistically proven value of certain management therapies in the group. It is also about what is best for the individual. Again, if this precept is forgotten I think we will create a terrible problem.

It would be quite improper to be in any way complacent. I do not honestly believe that most doctors are complacent concerning the current state of health care. I nevertheless think that the UK primary care system—our general practitioner training programme and the overall quality of our primary care doctors—is the envy of the world. I think there are few who would challenge that. Likewise, I think our schemes of clinical and applied research are certainly the envy of North America—and few would challenge that. The quality of our specialist training schemes and the opportunities afforded by the NHS are the reasons why North America appreciates what we can do in clinical research in which they have lagged behind. Both of these are crucially dependent on the training that we provide for our young doctors. It was Charles Lamb who said: 'Even judges were young boys once.' We should remember that every senior specialist and every experienced GP, on whom patients so heavily rely, was an undergraduate once. We ignore this point at our peril.

I also want to explain how education and research extends into every cell of the National Health Service. It is not something that can be 'bolted on' after the system had been put in place. Unless we really appreciate that we will get a completely wrong idea of the length and breadth of education and research. I want to get away from the rhetoric and the ideals and to say something about the reality of what is actually happening and what we really need. To highlight the perils so that we can be constructive and make sure that they are avoided.

All the issues I shall mention are only examples of the complementary locking together of education and research in the health care system of this country.

What will be the effect on teaching of case-mix changes of patients in the sorts of hospitals that Angela has just described? What will be the effect on teaching of separation of out-patient and in-patient services with much more procedures being performed on a day-stay and out-patient basis? What will the effect be on more formal teaching of rotating junior doctors to different hospitals in order to get experience in managing the full spectrum of diseases? Will shortened in-patient stay affect teaching and how can this be prevented? Will SIFT, the additional funding for the clinical costs of teaching in general but undergraduates in particular, really cover the costs? Will the teachers have the time? What effect will self-governing hospitals have on the academic career structure? These are all fundamental questions.

Education is not just about undergraduates of course; education is also about postgraduate and specialist training, the continuing education for the trained and the updating of teachers.

What about undergraduates? I would suggest that time in their training programme is absolutely crucial. The one word I would hope that you will take away from this talk is 'time'. Undergraduates need time to learn and practise their skills, particularly communication. We all know and admit that communication is far from satisfactory at present. They have to watch and experience history-taking and other aspects of the art of medicine that cannot be conducted in seminars or lecture theatres. They have to grasp the balance between the art and science of medicine, which of course is the essence of good practice. If we go too far towards the science, which is the easy aspect to teach, we shall lose the art and British medicine will be in disrepair. Undergraduates have to observe and be part of continuing care. All those subtleties, for example what a patient is like before and after an operation and the individual personal cost of that operation; not necessarily in financial terms, but in terms of their psyche and well-being. What about such issues as the 'four-day blues'? How do you teach an undergraduate that patients may be fine after they have just come round from an anaesthetic or from having a baby but that for many despair often comes when they are getting better, after three or four days. These are the subtleties of the art of medicine that we must not lose sight of and the students have to experience themselves. This is the apprenticeship side of medicine which I do not want to exaggerate nor do I want to ignore it either. Another teaching requirement is how to lead patients to the realization of serious implications: how do you tell a patient that they have a lethal illness? How do you help bereaved relatives? These are issues that students have to work through. They all require time and there is no substitute. Furthermore, they are very important for the quality of care that the White Paper is seeking. There has to be continuity for students to assess emerging investigations and new treatments. This is to allow them to learn to evaluate and discuss with their chiefs why they were used and whether it could be done more economically. If they do not have the continuity of observation they will not be there to see the problems.

Consider erosion of time and what may happen within the context of the White Paper. With emphasis on out-patients versus in-patients management, will the new structure of out-patients be such that it will allow time for teaching the undergraduates who have been transferred to out-patients because of the reduction in in-patients care? Continuity of learning and care may be very difficult when patients are coming up and being seen by different doctors on different occasions. It certainly will not be the same way as the old-fashioned ward round. Equally good alternatives may exist but they must be validated.

Again, to achieve some of the breadth of experience, rotations to peripheral hospitals will need to occur. But don't forget the travel time. Bill Hoffenberg mentioned this morning that his audit group met during the lunch hour. The students will not be there because they are travelling from one hospital to another. These are some very practical points. While you may solve one problem you very often create another, particularly in relation to education.

What about postgraduate education? Again, time is of the essence but the time requirements are obviously different. Studying and reading when so many junior doctors are over-tired or over-stretched is wasted time and we have to be aware of that. I am sure they should receive more supervision and formal instructions than they do at present. This is agreed by everybody but of course it requires time. That applies to both their general and specialist training. The postgraduates need to be kept in touch with basic sciences. Probably more so in the future than at present and this involves more structured time. They need to have time with consultants. These postgraduates are in training and it is no good us using them as service hands in out-patients unless they have the time to discuss their actions and management plans with the consultant. This at present is often very inadequate and I am not at all proud of what currently goes on in a lot of hospitals.

Again, let us consider this erosion of time. The doctors in training are working very long hours. One way of reducing the hours is to say that one doctor will cover more wards. This very often over-stretches the doctors that are on duty. They may be asked to cover disciplines which they are not really familiar with. That exaggerates their own anxiety when they are junior doctors in training. Consultant cover at the present time may be inadequate which again exposes the postgraduate trainees improperly to dangers and anxieties.

What about the trained? They need time for reading, discussing issues with the clinical team, and for teaching. They need time for proper preparation of that teaching, not 'blowing in and out', of which we have all been guilty. Counselling is of course also important. Then there are all these other duties—College activities, assisting the Department of Health, examining; all take consultants off site, often hundreds of miles away.

Let us consider the erosion of time for the consultants. With the changes in structure that have been suggested fewer junior staff may be on extended cover and may require more senior staff to cover the acute specialties. I've called it 'acting down'. This will lead to changes in patterns of work. Doctors, be they juniors or seniors, who are up all night, should have time to recover the following day if they are to perform adequately. The sleep-depriving rotas currently operative are incompatible with the high technology of acute medicine and must lead to a re-evaluation of current work patterns.

Overseas doctors were mentioned; perhaps 50 per cent in the registrar grade. Will they really be able to take on the same work as the career registrars? Certainly to begin with they may need considerably more supervision, both for their own sake as well as for the benefit of patients.

The management implications are obvious. The increased pressure of patient through-put entailed in contracts and the rationalization of services leading to out-lying clinics with doctors travelling between them will all generate practical problems. These are only some of the many practical difficulties that we will have to face. I have emphasized the crucial component of 'time' for the consultants, adequate cover for the juniors and adequate study time for all of them. Time, however, has to be translated into manpower. There is no way of avoiding this issue and this is where some of the excellent ideals of the White Paper have to be reconsidered in line with 'Achieving a Balance'. The manpower issue is a major problem which has not been tackled because of its obvious cost implications.

I was delighted to hear estimates for non-clinical consultant duties and that 45 per cent of a new consultant's time might be spent in non-clinical work. If the clinical work is going to be maintained at the same level and standard, which is obviously required, that could mean 45 per cent more consultants. And the cost of that..., I wonder? Clearly, new work patterns might help but the consultant expansion required is likely to be substantial.

Finally, I want to emphasize the range of clinical research. It is not just somebody going into a laboratory—as you well know. Research on cause and effect, includes research on risk factors in populations as well as laboratory studies on pathogenesis and disease mechanisms. Research to develop better methods of investigation must continue and a lot of research on treatment is needed. Research on prevention involves a multidisciplinary approach and are usually major studies. As a number of the managers very properly stressed, the natural history of many conditions has been quite inadequately researched in the past. Why? A major reason is because it is so difficult to maintain and fund these long-term studies.

Figure 12 shows how research permeates the whole structure of the community. There are three groups you can study: individuals with overt disease, those who have subclinical disease, and of course the healthy population. One

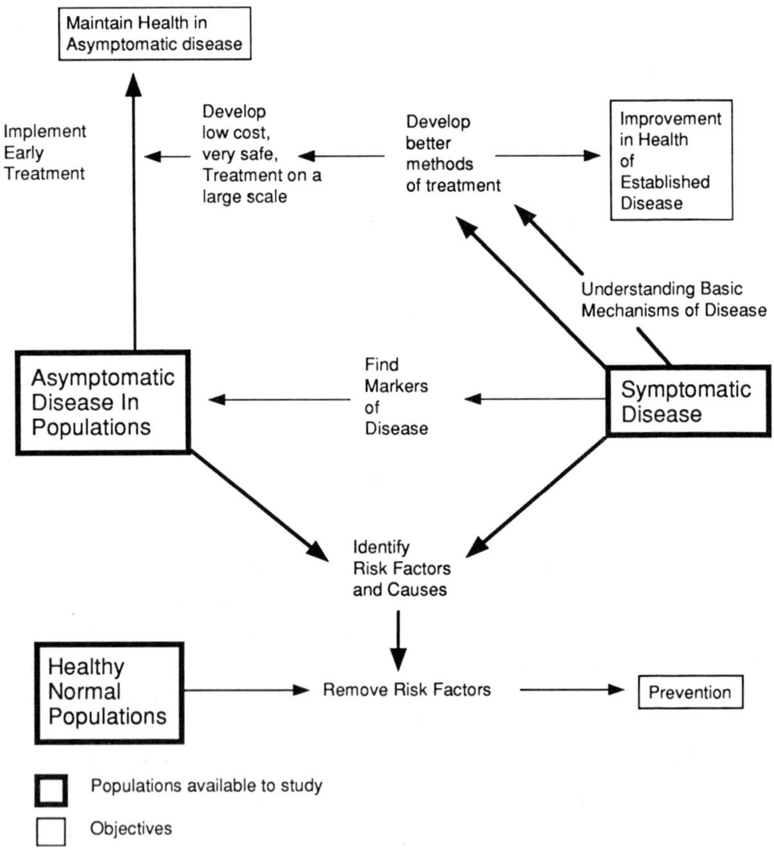

Fig. 12. The focus of research in respiratory medicine over the next ten years.

could argue that there has been much too much emphasis on investigating individuals with established disease, including understanding its causes, its pathogenesis, as well as developing better methods of treatment. All these types of research are necessary, as the investigation of these patients may define markers leading us to identify subclinical disease in apparently healthy people. Identification of alpha-1-antitrypsin deficiency first identified in some ill individuals, for example, will lead you to a group of healthy individuals who may some time in the future develop emphysema, particularly if they smoke. Thus investigating the group with overt disease can lead to the other groups in whom prevention may be possible. In order to start treating apparently healthy populations, the treatments have to be beneficial, of low cost, widely available and very safe. With early treatment those people who are fortunate enough not to have clinical symptoms may be maintained in a state which for all intents and purposes is healthy. Of course identification of risk factors, smoking and cholesterol screening for example, may enable one to modify the lifestyle in populations to keep them that way.

All these divergent types of research demonstrate the breadth of medical research, involving everyone... Work is progressing in all of these areas but there is a need for a much larger and more integrated effort. Against this background the severe cuts in Academic Medicine and National Councils support make no sense.

The variety and range of clinical trials need to be emphasized. These include small-scale clinical trials as well as large multicentre ones. Trials exist which explore new modalities of investigation, diagnosis, treatment, or prevention. Laboratory-based studies are only just one aspect of this spectrum of research. There are studies on the natural history of diseases as well as a huge range of epidemiological studies investigating prevalence, risk factors, and disease outcome. In order to perform these studies, we will need to identify suitable clusters of patient populations. They will be involved in additional attendances and probably longer in-patient stay with more investigations requiring additional personnel. That all means cost.

Lastly, Table 15 highlights the ramifications of modern multidisciplinary research, using breast cancer as an example. This type of research not only involves many medical and paramedical specialties, it leads to the development and implementation of specific treatment regimes as well as preventive screening programmes. So as soon as you take one important issue in medical practice, you find that very properly everyone is involved. Only in this way can we go forward, but it is extremely expensive.

Table 15: The importance of complementary studies as a research project, in this case breast carcinoma, is developed

The study	The specialty
Classification	Pathologist
Staging	Oncologist/radiologist
Hormone receptor sites	Pathologist
Hormone/chemotherapy treatment	Oncologist
Comparison with surgery	Surgeons
Management of secondaries	Physicians/Anaesthetists
Terminal care	Physicians/GP and team
Prevalence/risk factors	Epidemiologist
Screening programmes	Radiologist/team

In summary, these are some of the major hazards which we will have to face in the real world if teaching and research are to be maintained and expanded. Currently we have many structures in place which have been built up over the 40 years of the National Health Service. If we are to go forward, it will require both time and money. Great vigilance will be required to ensure that we will not go backwards.

14

The clinician–manager interface

MR DAVID KENNY

My immediate reaction to the title of this afternoon's address was to think of the 'BMA 5': consultant appointments committees, merit awards, consultant contracts, medical audit, and discipline. Five areas that have taken up a lot of time, emotion, and thought. Yet in a very real sense I think that the White Paper's arrival has radically widened the debate well beyond those specific issues. For example, it is of crucial importance to both the purchaser and provider functions in this new scheme that we rapidly achieve improved mutual understanding and commitment on the part of doctors and managers.

Taking the purchaser side as an example. If we are going to be creative in the specification of the service that the purchaser is trying to deliver, this really depends on a very sound and deep-rooted knowledge of just what is currently going on in medical development. This goes back to Margaret Turner-Warwick's comments on the need for informed support for research and teaching. A provider who does not get some good understanding and commitment from the consultants will not have a grasp of case-mix. If there is not an adequate grasp of case-mix in the provider, very soon—not necessarily immediately because we will start with block contracts—there will be the dangers of either over- or under-pricing.

For both purchaser and provider, unless there are clear programmes and targets for quality with real consultant and general practitioner commitment, we will be missing a very important part of the organizational cement. I do not mean quality as some nice optional add-on; I mean quality that is rooted in the procedures, tactics, and objectives of both parties.

You will not achieve this unless doctors are prepared to open up and have discussions that they have not had before with managers. Similarly, the managers need to be prepared to be much more explicit and proactive on the issues that they are confronting. I do see increasing scope for improvement and considerable improvement has already taken place. What I would like to do this afternoon rather than rely on exhortation and rhetoric, is to pick up some practical examples which we have come across in North West Thames. I will draw from two areas: first, my region's management development programmes for doctors; and secondly, some practical experience we have had with waiting lists.

As a preliminary, may I just observe that in our own view management development for doctors has relevance in four distinct contexts. Firstly, those doctors who want to take on full-time or near full-time management tasks, like UGM; secondly, those taking on responsibility for something like a medical directorate; thirdly, for those who really want to understand the management environment so that they can engage more successfully with the management of that institution; and fourthly, management techniques applied and aimed directly at the development of professional practice.

I do think that there remains a great deal of misunderstanding as to just what management is really about. This became very clear when Mr Roger Freeman took a very useful initiative last summer in suggesting that there should be some business school programmes for doctors. Now business school training for any manager is just a fragile phase in what is a very long-term process. The danger of the way in which Mr Freeman's initiative was seen in some quarters was that it really began to look like management training by sheep-dip. North West Thames as part of a consortium with a few other regions and the King's Fund, reacted to this by putting a counter-proposal to the Department of Health which has been selected. It specifies reasonably clearly, that there are three very important factors to take into account: preselection and preparation, the distinction between personal and management development, and follow-up support. I would just like to make a few comments about each.

First, preselection and preparation. Business schools will not accept from companies the 'problem children' who are causing disruption. As far as consultants are concerned, if a consultant—or in future I hope a general practitioner—is going on one of these programmes, he or she needs to be very clear why they are going. The business school, which is taking on this responsibility, really needs to be very clear why they are coming and both parties need to be very clear indeed about how success is to be judged.

The second point to be clear about is the difference between personal and management development. If we are going to talk to doctors about management development, to develop them either as clinician managers or as clinicians who can enjoy working with management more easily, then that development process must relate to the organization in which they work. The business school is just one part. They need to have formal support. The parties involved with the contract—the business school, the employer, as well as the clinician—need to be clear and committed to it. There needs to be a re-entry plan to make sure that the skills that they have picked up are actually employed and that they do not just subside into the same old patterns and feel demotivated.

The third part of this—the follow-up support—will require the existence of networks. We have found with our own consultant programmes, especially the early ones, that the people who had been on them were coming back to us and saying, 'Is there anybody else in this district or this hospital who has also been on this? I would like to talk to them.' And also, lessons learned from individual mentors—people who are prepared to help the person follow through some of these issues.

We have been running these consultant programmes for five years for all newly appointed consultants and it is a requirement on appointment that they join them. Two years ago we began programmes for senior consultants, and we have developed since then to new joint programmes where we are taking more risks. We are now running programmes for about 16 or 17 people. These include general managers, each with three or four consultants from their own district. Those joint programmes are beginning to produce even more practical results. We insist that practical, real issues are addressed and that they are then followed through. Development plans for clinical directorates, resource management, changes in paediatric services, are just a few of the themes that have been picked up and are now being followed through. What we want to see in the next few years is that this develops to working with general practitioners and hospital senior registrars and registrars.

I was talking to general practitioners recently about the new appointments of general managers in the FPCs. A very clear message coming through from them is an interest in management, displaying more open-mindedness than one might have been led to expect from some of the rhetoric. A very real anxiety exists that the new general managers might be coming from outside the Health Service and may act unthinkingly or not understand what they are doing.

I think my observation on the way in which the consultant programmes have developed is that the dialogue is now totally different. Originally when we started this off we had a presence in each programme of 14 or 16 consultants with two or three saboteurs. Over the last few years we have had none. Concurrently, the standard of questioning has become much more penetrating and the debate more open. Those who teach on it are having to work much harder which I think is healthy and good.

A second main area to draw from is our experience on waiting lists. The unit general managers who sat down some 15 months ago to address waiting list targets had varying degrees of success. Looking back at the results of the programmes of change that came out of it, it is now very clear that there was a sharp distinction between units with little tradition of clinicians and managers agreeing to common objectives and ways of working towards those objectives, compared to those units where the UGMs sat down with the clinicians, specialty by specialty, and bargained and traded so that both parties were learning about the real problems. For the former, it was a paper exercise, it was administration. It was a matter of issuing a policy statement with desirable targets, setting up some mechanism for reporting progress. But the targets were not negotiated with relevant clinicians, and therefore there was no ownership or commitment. Nor was there any detailed examination or real searching of the way in which the service was currently working and therefore no real change was likely to occur. For the latter group the targets were much more realistic, the action that followed was real and we got sound results out of it. That was management and it was joint management.

That has a spin-off effect. In Ealing, the surgeons have themselves, without being prompted, produced their own scheme for having a blitz on hernias and varicose veins. Their problem has been that these constituted a significant section of the waiting list and yet it is seen to be boring work. They have produced a scheme which actually deals with the boring part of the work without interfering too much with the more interesting work they want to do. This involved some reprogramming and some giving up of their time. It is, however, a scheme which is of their own making, it is acceptable to management, and is working well.

A different example of what is sometimes a very fragile interface, is audit. Now I think the posturing on both sides about access to information on this has not been helpful. I think there have been theological debates as to who owns the data, which is totally irrelevant. Both parties are on the same side. Managers want quality of care first and foremost and I do not accept the proposition from some of my general manager colleagues that the prerequisite is that they should have free and open access to all information. What I think the general manager needs to know is: first, that a system exists; secondly, that it is a system that identifies the problems; thirdly, that there is a mechanism to deal with those problems; fourthly, that this mechanism will be invoked by the profession when required; and fifthly, that if those measures fail, management will be given a full and timely account. Issues of discipline and competence must be addressed, but these will be more effectively addressed in the long term by keeping them in context. Until then, really the whole of the conduct of audit is to achieve results and quality. In the work that has been done in North West Thames Region the issues about who is going to have access to data just fade into the background as both sides get down to producing results and measurements of enduring improvement. The agenda has thus shifted from how do we get quality to how do we make sure it is sustained.

The standard of debate, while improving, every now and again displays signs indicative that the two cultures still have a lot to learn. I will just pick up two of those. One is in relation to management ethics or values. The management in a South Bedfordshire Hospital recently discharged a senior nurse manager who had repeatedly been arranging clinical tests for one of his children through his own and the laboratory staff. When he was discharged there was a protest from the local consultants who thought that the nurse manager really had not done all that much that was bad. As they saw it, he had used a few hospital materials. The point which the local management had considerable difficulty in getting across was that, by persistently using his own staff in something which was an improper practice, he had actually destroyed his own credibility as a manager of those nurses. They could no longer look upon that manager as someone who would act with integrity in a managerial context. That was something which the local management were right on but it needed much more explanation than had been appreciated for it to be understood by the local clinicians.

Not only does the interface between doctors and managers require further effort, but we also need to take a wider look at where we are in relation to the public. The *Sunday Times*' 'Insight' recently ran an item about consultants in private practice. We were interrogated by the 'Insight' team to see what our reaction was to the consultant physician who was at a private hospital when he was supposed to be, according to the out-patients' board, taking part in a clinic at his NHS hospital. Both I, the District General Manager, and the Director of Public Health were quite happy that this consultant's contract was properly completed. It was known that on Wednesday afternoons he was at the private hospital. This was by arrangement and for many years the NHS clinic had been conducted by registrars. That was not the answer that the *Sunday Times* was actually working towards. They quite rightly made the point, 'Well look: that is all very well, he may have been working to contract but the health authorities who are involved in this surely have a wider responsibility because the patient is expecting that there is a clinic with this chap's name above it and they expect to have a consultant in charge'. In that little episode, I think perhaps we lost sight of some of the wider issues involved in the debate about how the management and clinician interface is proceeding.

I think that essentially we are pointed in the right direction. We have made some good progress but it is rather like mountain walking. The result of climbing up the foothills is that you can actually see that there are a number of ways forward. What you also discover at the same time as you make such progress is that there is an awfully long way to go to the top, much longer than had appeared to be the case when looking up from the valley. So it will take time, we need sustained effort, but I think we can start now.

15

Discussion

Chairman: I think we have had three excellent, instructive, and certainly stimulating papers and now we have discussion. Discussion is, in my view, a two-way process and if you want to contribute as well as ask questions I think that is fine.

Dr Michael Joffe: I was very interested to hear Mr Kenny discuss the information coming out of audit and indicate that doctors and managers were on the same side. I think that has been true till now, but potential areas of conflict exist. When we are talking of the separation between providers and District Health Authorities, it is precisely on the quality of the care delivered and access to the audit figures that we are opening up a conflict of interests. I suggest we are not going in the right direction at all.

Mr David Kenny: What is the conflict of interest?

Dr Michael Joffe: Whether the contract will be renewed if the quality is deemed to be insufficient by the purchaser authority. That surely is the bottom line behind these reforms?

Mr David Kenny: I think that is nonsense in any other category. You do not get that approach by employers in ICI or Shell. They are very careful indeed when their research departments or their scientific staff have problems. People who are involved in developmental work—in work where there are no precise answers—are entitled to fail. The approach to handling the results of audit should be no different from those that are followed in other outstanding companies. The whole business of sacking people for fault is really a very remote possibility, and a great many steps are to be taken for somebody who has been found persistently unable to correct their performance over time, in spite of help from colleagues. There are all kinds of things that we do for medical staff at junior level that we should also be doing for consultants. It is beginning to happen and I think there is not enough open discussion about it. But to see audit as some kind of secret weapon is wholly folly. The more you see it related to quality and outcomes, the more confidence will be generated in its handling.

If a unit general manager started getting into some sort of macho disciplinary mood on audit in a region, that would be the end of good audit. It would have put paid to quality. So even if it were to take place in the way you have described it, it would have disastrous consequences.

Professor Margaret Turner-Warwick: Of course, mutual confidence is absolutely right and I agree with David. But take a simple example like wound infections. What I think the medical people want to do is to discuss openly and in confidence the frequency of their wound infections, to examine the worst cases, and perhaps to take some further swabs. This, in order to raise the standards. On the other hand, if wound infections are to be used as one of the criteria of obtaining a contract competitively with other hospitals, the way to reduce the number of wound infections would be to take no swabs! The medical people are saying that we need to identify and investigate the worst cases to raise standards and improve education. If that rebounds on the contracts, we have not served our managers or ourselves.

Dr Brian Seaton: A comment rather than a question. We seem to be falling into this trap again of seeing medical audit as an inquisitorial approach aimed at punishing failure. I think we should perhaps review the experiences of people like Chris Wyatt. In his book *Hospital-wide quality assurance*, he describes quality audit as being the primary process by which we will identify and reward quality. In chemical pathology, which is my area, the NECRAS Schemes were originally perceived in much the same kind of light: samples were sent out to labs in order to detect those which fail. Now the position is the reverse: the samples are sent out so that those labs which are successful can demonstrate their success and the people who use them can be confident in what is coming out of them.

Dr Sally Hargreaves: Listening to the first two speakers, I am really quite frightened about the future of the National Health Service. I cannot envisage anybody wanting to become a consultant who is on call one night in three, has 50 per cent managerial duties, is expected to be an expert in their specialty, as well as carrying out the mundane tasks previously undertaken by his junior staff. I wonder what the panel think.

Dr Angela Jones: I think you are actually painting a very gloomy picture. Consultants are on call now and my feeling is that we should be much more explicit about that. If there are fewer juniors then perhaps they will be on call in a more 'active front line' way and there will have to be compensations for that. We have to work in a reasonable way. For example, if you are on call one night then you will not be expected to do a heavy out-patient clinic the following morning.

What I was trying to say about other duties is that being a consultant doesn't just mean you are an expert in the clinical field. You are an expert in all the other hidden things as well; all are essential, for example, teaching, advocacy, and acting in the political arena. I think in the past consultants have not actually accepted these as their role; they thought of them as optional extras. I believe these are not additional but are part of being a consultant.

I think if all you want to do is the clinical work that you have just described, then you will not be a consultant—you will be something else, be it a staff grade or whatever.

Professor Margaret Turner-Warwick: I am glad that the issue of morale of junior staff has been raised because I do believe it is a very serious one. I have been very worried about the report of Isabel Allen which suggested that 44 per cent of junior staff actually were having second thoughts about continuing in the profession. The fact that so many are really disillusioned and depressed is very serious. That has been confirmed by a Manchester study looking at why medical students entered medicine. The challenge is through education to do much more for them and to take this opportunity of getting the conditions of service right. Otherwise it will go back to the sixth forms and there will be no more recruits.

Dr Peter Sheridan: Professor Turner-Warwick, I was very impressed with your slide of the number of people involved in the treatment of one condition—carcinoma of the breast. One of the things that worries me a lot about the White Paper is the move from a co-operative mode to a competitive mode. I just want to ask you: can the competitive mode be as comprehensive as the current co-operative mode? How can quality be guaranteed when competition comes in?

Professor Margaret Turner-Warwick: Thank you so much. I did not write the White Paper and I could not agree with you more. Over the last 10 years collaboration amongst the profession to get the very best out of the limited cash has been the operative mood. Collaboration exists between hospitals so that they do not duplicate services and work in the most economical way. We were just getting into a splendid mode of realistic collaboration and I think it is rather sad that we have been thrust into this alternative mood.

Professor Walter Holland: First of all can I thank our parent College for giving the prominence to our type of research. I am delighted that we have taught them something!

I have a question for each member of the panel, if we are concerned with research. I am concerned firstly at how in fact the manpower can be tailored to fit those doing full-time or part-time research, and how this is going to be fitted in, both during the training period as well as in the consultant grade. Secondly, I am very interested in the way in which the regional or the purchasing authorities will view and purchase research. Will they turn to proper research or continue to support management consultancy? And finally, I am very concerned at how in fact training for all forms of research can be sustained within competitive organizations.

Dr Angela Jones: I am sure Professor Holland knows that this problem of research, at what stage it is done in medical training, and how you tie up the numbers in academic departments and research departments with NHS training grades, is one that has been exercising the members of JPAC. I do not think anybody has yet come to a satisfactory answer and I do not think that I have an answer either. But it does seem to me that this is an inevitable problem when trying to develop manpower requirements in terms of career progression. There are restrictions on the number of research posts and that may have to be revised as the restrictions bite. I think it is a very serious problem and we have not yet come to a solution.

Mr David Kenny: I, for one, am very glad that this White Paper has not come out with instructions for use and a lot of detailed description. A lot of issues like research and development require the construction of some answers. We have to put some proposals forward, but there are no quick answers.

A point that is worth stressing concerns the nature of the competition. It will be managed competition, let there be no doubt about that. Progressively, if we are going to have quality, the RHA and the purchaser network will be working within some kind of regulatory framework. I cannot see that you can achieve any quality without collaboration and without an explicit commitment for research of all types that Professor Turner-Warwick was talking about, as well as practical development. We have to find ways of stitching these in. For the moment, there are no answers—and I think we have some work to do.

Professor Margaret Turner-Warwick: Perhaps we could go back for one moment to the carcinoma of the breast issue. Here you have the danger of a local hospital which has general surgeons who do mastectomies. You have the Guys' Oncology Research Unit trying to do all the sorts of things that I listed on that slide. But of course, for the reasons that I also listed, the costs differ between the two. The orthodox answer to this is that those two hospitals will be competitive because SIFT—this additional cost for teaching *and* research—will cover that. As we all know, this uplift from 75 per cent to 100 per cent sounds all right but the base-line was shifted. So in real terms this will in fact be a 2 per cent increase. How this 2 per cent increase is going to cover the whole differential of the cost of undergraduate teaching and the special requirements which we need for this as well as adequate research is questionable indeed. In point of fact, research is going to be really imperilled because in the short term it may not be able to compete. The yield of research is so much longer term.

Professor I.R. Cameron: I think my remarks are addressed to Dr Jones. I was sorry to see that her omnipotential consultant of the future did not have any time for research.

Dr Angela Jones: I am sorry that research did not appear on the list that flashed up. I do think that it is very important. One of the things that may well come out of the review of contracts proposed in the White Paper is that at last consultants will be able to negotiate real time to do research, an opportunity which they have not had in the past—and maybe also negotiate the resources that they need for this.

Dr D. Richardson: I wonder if I can bring up another aspect of doctors and the new Health Service that has been worrying me. It derives a little from what both Professor Turner-Warwick and Mr Kenny have said.

I do not think this is the place to go into the merits of GP budgets, but it clearly is quite contrary to any concept of proper medical conduct for me to be ordering a mastectomy. That is not what I do. I send a patient where appropriate to a specialist for that specialist's advice, which may or may not include a mastectomy. It may now also have to include a sum of money, but that may be for subsequent negotiation.

What bothers me more, and this is really an extension of the same thing, is that the purchaser/provider concept seems to me to be leading towards corporatism in our professional relationships. I may be in a position, either as budget holder or in adhering to my health authority's contracts, of really sending the patient to the health authority for treatment instead of to a named specialist. The consideration may be held by the health authority that all of those specialists in some particular topic are equal. I guess there isn't a clinician in this room who would believe that to be true. I wonder how Mr Kenny and Professor Turner-Warwick view this—whether they have any solutions to what I see as a way, in fact, of fundamentally changing the nature of the way that medical practice has gone on in this country.

Mr David Kenny: Thank you Dr Richardson! I really do not see that the referral mechanisms need either become totally corporatist or compartmentalized. I would make one passing observation about the compartmentalization. We find that a number of the waiting lists for care in routine conditions are unnecessarily long because the patients have been assigned to named individuals who have a queue. In the units where this has been explored properly with the consultants, this compartmentalization has been broken down and has resulted in a shorter wait. I do not think any strict idea of the GP always referring to a named consultant is going to stand up to organizational scrutiny in the long term. Nevertheless, I cannot see that the contracting system should put everybody into a pool regardless; I do not think the patients, the consumers are going to wear that. I do not see that it is a necessary part of the armoury of the purchaser to insist on it and a good provider unit is going to provide flexible systems so it can get round any sort of problem.

Professor Margaret Turner-Warwick: I think there is right on both sides. There may be some routine operations that most basic surgeons can do more or less equally well. When you come to the greyer areas of medicine then your point about different types of doctors for different types of patients applies. It may not only be quality, it may be that somebody is kinder or whatever. All sorts of different factors will come in making the best one-to-one match. If the GP knows the consultant is available he will try to make that fit.

There is one very fundamental issue that you raised about the purchaser/provider split and the GP's role that worries me. There is an excellent document that has just been written by the Royal College of General Practitioners on *Academic general practice: a strategy for academic practice*. In that, the authors have emphasized the continuum and partnership between the general practitioner and the consultant. The White Paper has plucked out the general practitioners and put them right over the other side in this purchaser role. This is a problem for the general practitioners—how are they going to sort out this tremendous dichotomy? I believe that general practitioners and consultants have to work very closely together and not allow themselves to be divided in this way.

Mr Jonathan Beacon: Mr Kenny, I just wondered about these opting-out hospitals. There is a pressure to see lots of hip patients, for example, who will be discharged quickly and we will get funding for our hospital from our general practitioners. Most of my patients who have hip operations are old people who stay in for a long time. Over 60 per cent of our beds are blocked for three to ten months for various reasons. Is there going to be pressure on consultants to seek 'more commercial-type surgery' in order to keep opted-out hospitals financially viable? Or will there be some mechanism for allowing us to maintain our service to the people who really need it?

Mr David Kenny: Could I use this opportunity to make a point about opting-out hospitals, subsequently called self-governing hospitals, and now called NHS trusts. It is this: in contracting terms from 1 April 1991, both the directly managed units and the NHS trusts will be operating on a contract basis. So any hospital will be competing for its income through the contracting system. There will not be a real difference over time between the directly managed and the self-governing units. In fact I think the self-governing units are there to break the mould and to create the split between purchaser and provider.

A second quick point. A few of us went over to the East Coast of the US and had a look at just the kind of problem that is being raised. The best way of getting good-quality care is to make sure that the purchaser is specifying in an innovative way and that the homework is done. Equally the provider also needs to be very much on top of the issues, such as case-mix, and to avoid problems inherent in going for short-term solutions. Now, the sort of example that you have given as a question is a short-term solution—a quick fix. Where that has been adopted in the US it has put the provider into difficulty. The arrangement presaged in the White Paper is that we should have rolling contracts looking three years ahead. That gives enough time for purchasers, who have got their wits about them, to get the balance of the specification in such a way that we can avoid the sort of problem which you raised.

Mr Anthony Richards: Dr Angela Jones has told us many of the factors that are weighing on the manpower equation and often pulling in different directions. I wonder if there may be another? The new purchaser, armed with the existent or non-existent data which have come from outcome measures and needs measures as discussed this morning, and able to use the money in non-hospital ways for health rather than for health services, may simply not purchase a certain specialty. I can see this as a possibility. If that is repeated several times this would alter the manpower equation. Is that so unlikely that it will not happen?

Dr Angela Jones: In theory I suppose it is a possibility. Taking your point a bit further, one of the problems with planning medical manpower is the length of time it all takes. I think we are going to witness some dramatic changes over the next five years where there may be different emphases within specialties when new needs are thrown up. We are not in any position with fairly tight controls to actually respond to that. I do not know what will happen. It makes it all very interesting and exciting!

Professor Margaret Turner-Warwick: This is a terribly important issue, because of course the 'Achieving a Balance' exercise and its formula was devised before the White Paper. The things that Angela and I were saying suggest that those numbers and that formula may be way out. Not a 2 per cent per annum increase for consultants, but 40 per cent. That may be an exaggeration, but it may be a difference of that order of magnitude.

The second thing that was not included in the formula was the assessment of need for the population, which District Health Authorities are now charged to do. When you scrutinize figures, such as 60 consultant cardiologists per million in the US compared to 6 per million in this country, part of it may be due to our different style of practice and primary care. When you have a difference of that order of magnitude, is it possible we are under-staffed? There is substantial factual evidence supposing that this formula may be seriously adrift.

Dr Wendy Sommerville: To follow on from my colleague orthopaedic surgeon who spoke before, I share his concerns. Consider what has happened in the US with DRGs. Patients who have hip operations are discharged early and they go to nursing homes. There are twice as many people who go to nursing homes, need long-stay care, and do not go back to the community again, compared to before DRGs were introduced. I have not seen any solution proposed as to how that should be dealt with.

Chairman: Thank you very much. We now have a change of scene. In introducing Professor Klein, I am sure he will not mind if I tell you where I first met him. It was 1975 and we were attending a great seminar on *One year on*—it was one year after the 'Grey book' on which I served and he criticized. We had then the great new panacea of all medicine: consensus management. It was untried, it was untested, it was unproven, and in the end it was unworkable! So that is where we first met, and I am dying to hear how we are going to take the issues forward this time round.

16

Taking the issues forward
(or: Taking the issues backwards)

PROFESSOR RUDOLF KLEIN

When one is asked to sum up a conference it is too tempting to refuse: one doesn't have to prepare anything. All one has to do is just send in a long CV to fill the space where other speakers have put a summary. However, during the course of the day one begins to feel a sense that one might possibly have taken the wrong decision! Particularly I think at a conference like this where the contributions have been of such a high standard. If I were to attempt to sum them all up and bring them together in a nice tidy way, I am afraid all of you would not only miss your glasses of sherry but also your trains home.

So I decided on a slightly different tack. This saves me from having to get in the obligatory reference to each and every speaker and from having to make sure, like a party political broadcast, that each of the previous speakers gets exactly the same amount of summing up time. What I have decided to do is to imagine myself at a conference in the year 2000 organized by Dame Sheila Adam, as she is by then, to celebrate the tenth anniversary of this conference: to look back on this conference with the benefit of hindsight and talk about the printed version of everybody's papers.

Here I am speaking or probably croaking, this frail figure having been wheeled on in a wheelchair and requiring a bit of sympathy from the audience, looking back on this conference and remarking in retrospect how surprisingly gloomy the whole atmosphere was. Analysing the contributions—including those from the floor—a remarkable division between the managers and the medical contributors was apparent. The managers on the whole stressed the opportunities and the doctors all stressed the problems ahead. I didn't keep a systematic tally, but I think in retrospect you will see that this in fact was the case.

Now you might cynically react by saying, 'Well, of course: absolutely natural. What the White Paper does is to create the opportunities for managers and problems for clinicians.' That might be one possible reaction. I am going to suggest that this might be an over-simplification. You will realize that I am now speaking from the point of view of the year 2000 with hindsight and all that entails. I think we often fall into a curious psychological trick: the trick is to invent both an imaginary past when all was well and an imaginary future when all the problems came up.

Let me illustrate this in the light of our discussion this morning, particularly concerning the problems of information required to make need assessment possible and the lack of available information required for financial management. It was very moving, I felt, that great lament about all this extra information which we will require in order to make the new system work. However, it did irreverently cross my mind, well it rather crossed my mind in the year 2000, what an extraordinary indictment that actually is of the system with which we have been living for the last 40 years. If now suddenly, in the year 1990, we start saying that we haven't really got the basic information for making the Health Service run properly, some future historian may well say that whatever the risks and the element of gamble involved in the 1989 White Paper, it was actually better than perpetuating a status quo which in many important respects had failed to deliver.

We can illustrate this in fact and, Chairman, you anticipated me on this. One of the difficulties I have going to conferences these days is that doctors are getting younger the whole time, especially public health physicians. I am therefore never quite sure how far back their memories go, but the Chairman helped me by already drawing your attention to the 1974 reorganization of the NHS. It is interesting from our current perspective, that this time round everybody is arguing about the way the government precipitated and rushed into change without proper consultation. It was all done by Downing Street and even the Department of Health at times did not know what was going on. Now look at 1974. As the Chairman has already indicated, from many points of view, it was an absolute model of how to get change done. At least we thought so at the time. Endless consultation—Sir Keith Joseph in those days was the greatest corporatist of them all. The principle on which the 1974 reorganization was carried out that one no one should be able to disagree with. Everybody was so smothered in committees that in the end, out of sheer boredom and weariness, they all agreed. Great investment in training, endless preparation, conferences, meetings, and so on. Yet, as the Chairman rightly said, disillusion followed very quickly.

Take one particular example. The discussion this morning rightly emphasized that the driving force behind the purchaser/provider relationship should be needs assessment of the population. Relax—I am not going into the theology or concept of 'need'. All I am going to do is remind you that this was precisely the emphasis of the 1974 reorganization. If you look at Keith Joseph's preface to the Green Paper or the Grey Paper, it said that Health Service planning should start from the basis of looking at the needs of the population. Now, this did not happen and certainly this morning, I at times got a sense of 'I've been here before'—all the same arguments.

That leads one to ask: what in fact, if anything, is different about the 1989 White Paper which might lead one to expect by the year 2000 a more successful outcome? I think in fact there are some differences. The new idea of the provider/purchaser relationship actually does introduce some incentives to managers to develop this idea of assessing what the 'needs' or 'demands' of a given population are. A further big difference this time is that there is actually going to be a major investment in the infrastructure of management. I do think the Government has been pushed into this rather than anticipating it. Now if you go back to 1974, as the Chairman said, that was rapidly overtaken by oil crises, inflation, economic crises, and cuts in NHS management. Public sector manpower—some of you may remember—suddenly became a bad thing. One of the reasons why the 1974 reorganization failed was in fact that there was never the build-up of managerial and epidemiological expertise required to make it work.

This time we will find that there is going to be a quite massive infusion of extra managerial and epidemiological man- and womanpower. If you look at the appendix to the National Health Services and Community Care Bill you will see that there is actually provision for an extra 3000 posts—posts ranging from finance personnel and information technology staff at the hospital and regional level. The regions won't have any excuse for not appointing splendid researchers and epidemiologists.

Another big difference is that we really have learned a great deal in the intervening 15 or so years about what planning is. If you go back to the 1970s, planning was all about drawing up those great shopping lists. Planning was seen in terms of inputs: if you wanted to increase services, we needed extra doctors, nurses, and all the rest of it. The shopping lists were endless and all the Government's priorities, White Papers, and so on, saw the achievement of priorities in terms of achieving certain manpower/womanpower inputs. I think what we have learned now—and this came up this morning—is that planning is essentially opportunistic. You have to be quite clear about where you want to go and about your basic aims, but how you get there is an experimental and opportunistic process. You take your chances in good years when the Treasury has given you lots of money, perhaps because an election is about to come, and you can expand. In bad years you make do. So we actually have learned a lot about how to set about this.

Hence, my hunch is that in ten years' time when we are looking back, we will think that the optimists on the whole were more right than the pessimists. The great reorganization wasn't such a big deal after all and, curiously enough, things went on in not all that different a way. There were all these block contracts with hospitals and those hospitals operated as they had done before. A gradual change in both the clinical and managerial culture began; but even ten years later all these things were still in the process of working themselves through. The great political drama which introduced all these changes has given us a deceptive sense of being in the middle of a great revolution. In retrospect, I think, 1989 will not be *the* revolution of the National Health Service, but just another interesting staging post in its continued evolution.

Let me now turn to some of the specific issues raised at that interesting conference organized in 1990 and look at how we might reflect on some of those. I didn't say so at the beginning, but I quickly changed the title of my talk to 'Taking the issues backward'! So taking the issues backward, what might we reflect on the specific points raised today?

I think in about 1995 an American will have published a book called *The selling of the DRG*. In it he will point out the large investment made by management consultancies and others in selling cross-nationally the DRG—the Health Service equivalent of 'Coca Cola'—to everybody. Then will come the story of disillusionment with it. In fact if you read the study carried out by Harvey Sapolski and his colleagues at MIT into what happened in New Jersey where DRGs were first tried out, it already indicates a certain note of caution. I perhaps ought to have confessed at the beginning, that my record in making predictions tends to be patchy at best. A year or two ago I was assuring Americans that the British would never be idiotic enough to fall for the DRGs, since I didn't see that they had very much application in this country. So my predictions for the year 2000 will have to be taken with a certain reserve. One can never account for people's credulity!

Taking some of the other retrospective reflections, I think the conference in the year 2000 will still be scratching its head about the question of outcomes. Again, somebody by then will have written *The history of the search for outcomes* and will have pointed out that the problems had been around a long time already in the year 1990. Maybe at that time they should not have been all that optimistic about this as a 'tin opener' for assessing need.

At the same time, there may be an increasing amount of scepticism about using population health outcomes as targets for health authorities. I think some regional managers may by then have discovered that they went into this perhaps a touch too eagerly and found that a lot of the factors which actually decided health outcomes were beyond their control. I think that is a basic problem. By then of course you will have had the famous schism with the 'pope' of the NHS moving to Leeds therefore creating problems for the rest of the 'church' left in London. I think the interesting split that may occur at that particular point is that the London part of the 'church' will decide to put its future in arguing with the rest of Whitehall about other forms of policy making with an implication for health. It will be left to the 'pope' at Leeds simply to run a Health Service; a nice, good garage service for people like me, who simply want to take their bodies in to be repaired when they need it and who are interested in the way they are treated rather than in population outcomes.

Now moving on from that to information systems. I suspect that looking back in ten years' time there will be some degree of surprise at the narrow way in which the debate on information systems was conducted in the year 1990. That the debate didn't revolve, as by the year 1993 it already was revolving, about linking hospital and general practice data. After all, this is probably the only way of getting the longitudinal information which you need if you are going to look at efficacy over time and not just three days after the patient leaves hospital. I think, too, there will be retrospective criticism of the Government for investing very heavily in general practitioner information systems without using this as an incentive for them to develop systems compatible with the hospital sector. Equally there will be some surprise at the narrow definition of information needs and the exclusion of getting information about what the private sector is doing. Yet if, for example, you look at population needs in terms of demands, as somebody was suggesting this morning, then surely the one place where you actually get a lot of information about unsatisfied demand is the private sector. In fact, of course, in the year 2000 we will find that it was the minority Labour Government of 1996 which passed legislation making it compulsory for the private sector to provide information about its activities to the NHS planners.

Looking back in the year 2000, we will probably find experiments, like joint purchasing authorities between health and social and local authorities, proliferating. That seems precisely the kind of experimental approach likely to emerge from all the anguish at the moment. We will also look back with surprise at the issues which were not discussed at all. The one which surprised me most of all—particularly with Dr Marks as Chairman—was the implications of a possible change in the balance of roles between GPs and consultants. One of the things where I was wildly wrong when the White Paper came out concerns the idea of GP budgets. I thought you needed a much larger managerial infrastructure than an 11000 patient practice could provide. I think I was totally wrong about that. Now, given the sort of enthusiasm I sense out there, the implications are extraordinarily far reaching. There are obvious implications for the budgets of the health authorities. They will soon start looking like those mints advertised on television; there will be a large hole in them. A hole which the general practitioners will bite out as they go for budgets. Locally, I heard of one general practice which intends to use its budget to hire consultants to hold their out-patient clinics in the GP's surgery. Now that seems to me to be a highly attractive idea from the point of view of patients. Imagine the implications if that sort of thing spreads. I can see quite significant changes and a diffusion of power away from the health authorities and the hospital sector towards primary health care. Very interesting, but it obviously complicates all the things we have been discussing, such as planning for meeting particular needs. If you have got this sort of plurality of buyers who collectively will have a quite formidable purchasing power, what does this in fact then do? Again, I am looking forward to the sort of problems which will emerge in ten years' time rather than now, but I think we ought to be aware of them.

A theme throughout the day has been the movement towards explicit objectives and explicit rationing. Now, that could be extraordinarily destructive of the kind of cosy political cocoon which has surrounded and protected the Health Service. The Health Service has always rationed—we know that—but the rationing has never been explicit. It has been dissipated, dissolved, and made invisible by largely being left to individual clinicians. What happens in fact if—with this new policy of drawing up splendid documents, making it all explicit and actually deciding priorities—it becomes clear that we have decided not to do certain things?

The same kind of problems are going to come out with medical audit. Will we be able, on a long-term basis, to separate medical audit from resource management? It is all very well getting enthusiastic about quality, but quality is not an absolute and it costs money. Are we actually going to decide that quality is simply something we are going for, full stop? Or are we going to put a price on quality? Are we going to say, 'OK. This is good average quality and we will pay the price for that. We are not going to go for the top 20 per cent of quality'? In which case, can we separate analysis of resource management from analysis of quality through medical audit? Or will the two in fact at one point have to meet?

In conclusion, let me now just explain, Chairman, why Dame Sheila actually called the conference in ten years' time. Partly it was to mark the unveiling of the statue to Sir Kenneth Clarke—as he is by then—at what, by then, is the Royal College of Public Health Physicians. By the year 2000, everybody will have realized that whatever was right or wrong about the 1989 White Paper, it was an absolute bonanza for the public health physicians. They have never looked back since. Relieved from being entangled in the daily management of hospitals, no longer having to spend their time dealing with irate consultants and so on, public health physicians were actually able to do what the 'parents' of the profession always thought they should do: think grand thoughts about the planning of the National Health Service.

The other reason for the conference in the year 2000 is to look at the implications of the White Paper published by the then Labour Government for the future of the National Health Service. Let me quickly recall some of the history leading up to that particular event. The period 1990–92 turned out to be absolute boom years for the National Health Service. The Conservative Government, realizing the unpopularity of its reform measures, spent money lavishly on the National Health Service. You can already see some of the effects of this in the

Public Expenditure White Paper published today: a 3·4 per cent increase in real terms. This went on year after year.

Then came a period of minority governments, first Conservative, then Labour, where the balance of power in the House of Commons was held by the Scottish Nationalists. What happened then was that the National Health Service got starved of funds, but Scotland developed the best Health Service in Europe!

Then you had a period of Labour Government under the 'Iron Chancellor' as Mr Smith became known. In trying to deal with yet another economic crisis he just relied on the internal growth monies. These were generated by the efficiencies created by the 1989 White Paper proposals. This inevitably led to a major crisis whereupon Mr Kinnock appointed yet another working party to look at the funding of the National Health Service. Labour Governments are always advised by Hungarian economists, as you well know, and by the year 2000 the Hungarian economists were advising a market economy of health care. In fact the proposal was to hand over the funding and everything else to competitive insurance schemes. Mind you, they were non-profit-making insurance schemes, but they were going to be competitive. It was, Chairman, for that conference that we all assembled to consider, in retrospect, what this conference was about.

Chairman: If I can bring her down to earth, would Dr Adam please come and close the meeting.

Dr Sheila Adam: I suppose I should say, 'See you back here in ten years' time.' I think the damehood might be a little inappropriate, if not premature. I have enjoyed this birthday party today and I am always keen to organize more parties, so perhaps we will think about it in ten years' time. Thank you all very much indeed.

Contributors: biographical details

Sir Donald Acheson, KBE DM DSc FRCP FFPHM FFOM
Chief Medical Officer, Department of Health

Sir Donald succeeded Sir Henry Yellowlees as Chief Medical Officer on 1 January 1984. He has led the UK delegation to the World Health Organization (WHO) since that date and was Chairman of the WHO Committee for Europe in 1986–87. In May 1988 he became the UK member of the Executive Board at WHO.

A graduate of Oxford University (1951) his interest in the epidemiology of disease and the organization of health services is reflected in numerous publications on both subjects. His previous appointments include Founding Director, the Oxford Linkage Study (1960), Founding Dean and Professor of Clinical Epidemiology, the Medical School, Southampton (1968) and first Director, the Epidemiology Unit, MRC (1978) where he studied the identification of environmental carcinogens. He was a member of the Royal Commission on Environmental Pollution (1979–83) and has advised Government and MRC on problems including asbestos and lead in the environment.

Sir Donald chaired both the DHSS Working Group on Primary Health Care in Inner London and the Nuffield Trust Enquiry into the Care of the Elderly in 1980–81. He recently chaired the Public Health Enquiry, the report of which, *Public Health in England* (January 1988), presents the first major review of the public health function since the Royal Commission of 1871.

Dr Sheila Adam, MD FFPHM MRCP
Public Health Director, North West Thames Regional Health Authority

Sheila Adam was appointed Public Health Director for North West Thames RHA in February 1989. She is a medical graduate of the University of Edinburgh (1972) and trained in public health medicine in Oxford. She worked as a Specialist in Community Medicine in Brent Health Authority and then at North West Thames Regional Health Authority. Dr Adam was previously a member of the Board of the Faculty of Public Health Medicine and an elected member of the General Medical Council.

Dr Eddy Beck, MBBS, BMedSci, MSc, MFPHM
Senior Registrar in Public Health Medicine, North West Thames Regional Health Authority

Born in Indonesia of Dutch parents, Eddy Beck settled in the Netherlands at the age of five. Ten years later he migrated to Australia where he completed his secondary schooling and graduated at Monash Medical School. He subsequently returned to Europe to continue his postgraduate education. His appointment as Guy's Hospital's representative on the European Exchange Scheme in Medicine for Junior Doctors took him back to the Netherlands albeit in a professional capacity. Following this appointment he was employed as a registrar by North West Thames RHA and is currently an Honorary Clinical Lecturer in the Academic Department of Public Health, St Mary's Hospital Medical School. His areas of interest include infectious diseases epidemiology, developing information systems, and health services organization.

Professor Walter W. Holland, MD FRCP FFPHM
President, Faculty of Public Health Medicine

Walter Holland succeeded Dame Rosemary Rue as President of the Faculty of Public Health Medicine in June 1989.

His interest in the epidemiology of respiratory diseases and health services organization is reflected in numerous publications on these subjects. He is currently Professor of

Clinical Epidemiology and Chairman of the Division of Community Health at the United Medical and Dental Schools of Guy's and St Thomas's Hospitals. He is also President of the International Epidemiological Association.

Dr John Marks, MD FRCGP DObstRCOG
Chairman of Council, British Medical Association

John Marks was Chairman of Council BMA between 1984 and 1990. A graduate of the University of Edinburgh, he became a Principal in General Practice, Borehamwood in 1954 where he continues to practise as a general practitioner. His publications reflect both his clinical and managerial involvement with General Practice.

In addition to his clinical commitment he has been a member of a large number of local and national committees including a large number of previous BMA appointments.

Professor Rudolf Klein
Centre for the Analysis of Social Policy, University of Bath

Rudolf Klein was born in 1930 in Czechoslovakia and came to Britain in 1939. After a peripatetic education at a variety of schools he ended up at Merton College, Oxford. There he specialized in medieval history. From Oxford, he went to Fleet Street. He initially wrote leading articles at *The Evening Standard* and *The Observer*. Subsequently he became editor of the leader pages and home affairs editor at *The Observer*. In the early 1970s he moved from journalism to research. After a spell at the London School of Hygiene and Tropical Medicine which introduced him to health service research, he moved to the Centre for Studies in Social Policy as Senior Fellow.

In 1978 he moved on to become Professor of Social Policy at Bath University where he founded (and is Director of) the Centre for the Analysis of Social Policy. At Bath he, together with Patricia Day, developed the study of the public regulation of private welfare. This has included a study of the regulation of nursing homes, both in this country and in the United States.

He has written a number of books on the Health Service and has also written extensively in the *British Medical*

Journal, the *Millbank Memorial Fund Quarterly*, the *Journal of Health Politics, Policy and Law*, *Political Quarterly*, *Health Affairs*, *Political Studies* and the *British Journal of Political Science*.

Dr Greg Parston, PhD
Director, Office for Public Management, London

Greg Parston is a Director of the Office for Public Management, an institute which contributes to the development of theory and practice in the field of public management. He has worked as senior manager, consultant, and educator in several countries. His appointments have included management posts in New York State and in the Province of Ontario, as well as a residency with the US National Science Foundation. He has been a consultant to national and local governments, and numerous health, housing, education, voluntary, and professional agencies. Initially educated in economics and architecture, he did a PhD at University College London and has taught there as well as on the Faculty of New York University and the King's Fund College. He has written widely in the areas of public management, strategic management and planning, and management development.

Dr Deirdre Cunningham, MRCSLRCP DObstRCOG MSc MFPHM
Director of Public Health, Parkside Health Authority

Deirdre Cunningham was appointed to her current post in 1986 and is currently on secondment to the Department of Health. A graduate of the Royal Free School of Medicine she initially worked as a Principal in General Practice until 1981. Her subsequent public health medicine career involved working in Medway Health Authority, as a Lecturer in the Academic Department of Community Medicine, St Thomas's Campus, UMDS, and she has worked as a Specialist in Community Medicine in West Lambeth Health Authority prior to taking up her current post. She has recently been increasingly involved with developing the Public Health role in assessment of needs in collaboration with representatives from other districts.

Sir Raymond Hoffenberg, KBE MD PhD FRCP
President, Wolfson College, Oxford University

Sir Raymond is a graduate of the University of Cape Town (1948). He has published a large number of papers on endocrinology and metabolism and also has a longstanding interest in medical audit. He initially worked as a Senior Lecturer in the Department of Medicine, University of Cape Town from 1955 until his ban by the South African Government in 1967. He emigrated to the UK in 1968 and took up the post of Senior Scientist at the MRC. In 1972 he became the William Withering Professor of Medicine, University of Birmingham. He is a member of a large number of scientific societies and was President of the Royal College of Physicians from 1983 till 1989. His appointment at Wolfson College commenced in 1985.

Dr John Mitchell, MBBS MRCP
Visiting Fellow, King's Fund College

John Mitchell joined the King's Fund College in April 1988. He is on secondment from Waltham Forest Health Authority and North East Thames Regional Health Authority. There he had a dual role as Consultant Physician with responsibility for elderly people and General Manager of the Community Services Unit. Prior to 1985 he had been the Consultant Member of the District Management Team. He has extensive experience, both as a clinician and a manager in health care delivery and is particularly interested in the provision of quality services for elderly and disabled people. At the College he is responsible for co-ordinating management development programmes for doctors, is working with a number of health authorities in the introduction of resource management, contributes to a number of initiatives in community strategies, as well as having a continuing involvement in services for elderly people. He has spoken extensively on these and other issues and has a number of publications on quality and services for elderly people. He is a member of the Editorial

Board of the *Journal of Management in Medicine* and chairs ADA, a voluntary organization for people with dysphasia.

Professor Lou Opit, MBBS BSc FRCS FRACS FFPHM
Professor of Community Medicine, Centre for Health Services Studies, University of Kent

Lou Opit graduated from the University of Adelaide in 1949. He initially worked as a surgeon in both the UK and Australia, culminating in his appointment as Reader in Surgery, University of Adelaide in 1964. Prior to this appointment he spent a year at Harvard as a Harkness Fund Fellow.

He completed a degree in pure mathematics at Warwick University in 1969 following which he made a career switch to Health Services Research. His subsequent career included working as a Senior Research Fellow, Department of Social Medicine, University of Birmingham, and he became Professor of Social and Preventive Medicine at Monash University, Melbourne in 1976. He returned to the UK in 1985 to take up his current post and was Director of the Health Services Research Unit until 1988. Since coming to Canterbury he has also been involved with the Policy and Research Division of South East Thames RHA as well as acting in a regular consultancy capacity for WHO, Geneva. He has published extensively in the fields of surgical practice, biomedical, and health services research.

Professor Tony Culyer
Department of Economics and Related Studies, University of York

Tony Culyer is the Head of the Department of Economics at the University of York. He has previously taught at the University of California in Los Angeles and at Exeter University. He has held visiting professorships at Queen's University, Canada; the Ontario Economic Council, Canada; the University of Otago; the Australian National University; and at Trent University, Canada. He has published on many economic aspects of social policy, and has written many articles and books on health services. His next book will be a two volume edited collection of major articles in health economics to be published by Edward Elgar in 1990.

His entry in *Who's Who* cites church music as his principal activity outside economics: he is organist and choirmaster at a Yorkshire parish church and chairman of the York area of the Royal School of Church Music, and in his spare time has built a 'Regal' and a small pipe organ. Were his wife and children less committed to musical activities than they are they would see more and hear less of him.

Mr Alasdair Liddell,BA DMS LHSM
Regional General Manager, East Anglian Regional Health Authority

Alasdair Liddell has been Regional General Manager for the East Anglian Regional Health Authority since October 1988. His NHS career started in 1972 and has been concentrated in London until his move to Cambridge. Previous appointments include District General Manager, Bloomsbury Health Authority (1984–88), District Administrator for Hammersmith and Fulham Health Authority (1982–84), and a variety of more junior posts in central London at hospital and district level. He has a law degree from Balliol College, Oxford, a DMS from Thames Polytechnic, and has attended the Executive Programme at the London Business School.

Professor Elaine Murphy, MD FRCPsych
Professor of Psychogeriatrics, United Medical and Dental Schools, Guy's and St Thomas's Hospitals

Elaine Murphy has been Professor of Psychogeriatrics at the United Medical and Dental Schools of Guy's and St Thomas's Hospitals since 1983. Her main research interests are in the epidemiology of mental disorders in old age, especially depression and service evaluation studies.

She was seconded as District General Manager of Lewisham and North Southwark Health Authority and lead DGM for the South East London Commissioning Consortium of three teaching districts from 1988 to 1990. She is also Vice Chairman of the Mental Health Act Commission.

Dr Angela Jones, FFPHM
Consultant in Public Health Medicine, North West Regional Health Authority

Since 1985 Angela Jones has been responsible for all aspects of medical manpower planning and staffing in the Region.

Work undertaken includes:production of medical manpower strategy; proposals for safety net for districts, papers on the safety net by specialty for submission to the Department of Health; guidance for the reduction of junior doctors' hours; and proposals for rotations and definition of registrar.

Dr Jones has worked as a Specialist in Community Medicine in Kensington, Chelsea, and Westminster Area Health Authority and as District Medical Officer in the Victoria Health Authority prior to taking up her current post. She is Chairman of the English Regions Medical Manpower and Staffing Group, as well as a member of the Standing Committee on Medical Postgraduate Education, National JPAC, the Technical Sub-Group for Achieving a Balance, and the Joint Monitoring Group for Achieving a Balance.

Professor Margaret Turner-Warwick, MA DM PhD PRCP FRACP FACP FFOM
President, Royal College of Physicians

Margaret Turner-Warwick graduated from University College Hospital Medical School and became a Senior Lecturer, Institute of Diseases of the Chest in 1963. This followed her appointment as Consultant Physician, Elizabeth Garrett Anderson Hospital in 1960 and she was appointed Consultant Physician, the London Chest Hospital in 1967. She became Professor of Medicine (Thoracic Medicine) and Director, Department of Thoracic Medicine, Cardiothoracic Institute in 1972 and subsequently Dean of the Cardiothoracic Institute in 1984.

She has held a large number of elected and nominated appointments on both scientific and policy bodies, has written numerous scientific papers, and presented lectures and contributions to specialist symposia throughout the world. In 1989 she was elected President of the Royal College of

Physicians while continuing to work as Consultant Physician at the Brompton Hospital and Emeritus Professor of Medicine (Thoracic Medicine) at the National Heart and Lung Institute.

Mr David Kenny, LLB FHSM
General Manager, North West Thames Regional Health Authority

David Kenny was appointed General Manager to the North West Thames Regional Health Authority in 1984, having been the Regional Administrator since 1982. His post immediately before that date was Area Administrator of Kensington, Chelsea, and Westminster Health Authority (Teaching), having previously been District Administrator of Tower Hamlets Health District and House Governor of The London Hospital.

David Kenny is a Member of the National Council of the Institute of Health Services Management and was President of the Institute 1981–82. He was Chairman of the Data Protection Working Group of the International Medical Informatics Association from 1979 to 1987 and has published articles on data protection in health information systems and on management topics.

Contributors to discussions

Index